Special Praise for
Connecting in the Land of Dementia

"A 'must read' for every care partner because it really helps you to look at things differently! This book is very special in the way it provides you with hundreds of suggestions on how to be a good care partner for someone with dementia and enjoy this yourself as well. Deborah inspired me by bringing together so many positive examples of using creativity to engage with people with dementia."

Marc Wortmann
Executive Director, Alzheimer's Disease International

"'Making the most of the moment' is the essence of *Connecting in the Land of Dementia*. Deborah's creative and imaginative ideas on ways to engage your loved one with Alzheimer's disease are meant to channel frustration into fulfillment and lift the human spirit."

Meryl Comer
President, Geoffrey Beene Foundation Alzheimer's Initiative
Author of *New York Times* best seller *Slow Dancing with a Stranger: Lost and Found in the Age of Alzheimer's*

"With interesting, delightful, specific detail, the reader is shown how to keep the person living with dementia a part of life. Whether it is through art or gardening or storytelling or dancing or music, a life can go on. Bravo to Deborah Shouse."

Trish Vradenburg
Cofounder, UsAgainstAlzheimer's
Cofounder, WomenAgainstAlzheimer's

"*Connecting in the Land of Dementia* is a lively and essential guide for any dementia care partner who wants to help a loved one feel joy and purpose through simple, fun activities. It's also a rare collection of wisdom from dozens of experts worldwide who specialize in creative dementia care. We can turn to any chapter and be inspired."

Martha Stettinius
Author of *Inside the Dementia Epidemic: A Daughter's Memoir*

"Buy this book, read it, highlight what inspires you. As you make notes and bend pages to personalize this guide, you are creating a family treasure."

Carol Bradley Bursack
Founder of Minding Our Elders

"*Connecting in the Land of Dementia* is an inspiring and creative compilation of activities for dementia caregivers. Even longtime healthcare professionals will find innovative new projects to add to their routines. We should thank Shouse for her lovingly prepared collection that will be indispensible to so many of us."

Sandra Stimson CADDCT CALA, AC-BC, ADC, CDP, CDCM, CFR-DT
CEO, National Council of Certified Dementia Practitioners

"Deborah Shouse provides a great public service by shining light on the numerous creative activities that can meaningfully engage the minds and spirits of persons living with dementia. From personalized music to storytelling, Shouse makes it easy for caregivers to understand the various options they have to help their loved ones navigate through their everyday lives."

Dan Cohen, MSW
Founding Executive Director, MUSIC & MEMORY[SM]

"Once again, Deborah Shouse delivers a book that softens our hearts and opens our minds to find fun ways to connect to the soul. No matter what our situation in life, no matter what our ability is to communicate, we all crave and need to be connected to one another."

Lori La Bey
Radio Host, Keynoter, and Founder of www.alzheimersspeaks.com

"*Connecting in the Land of Dementia* simply shines as a beacon of hope for persons living with dementia and their care partners. There's at least one great idea on every page. I highly recommend it."

Mara Botonis
Author of *When Caring Takes Courage*

"Deborah has created an assuring, light of heart and deep in wisdom weaving of the great thinkers and practitioners in the field of dementia care. Here you will find bite-sized, inspirational approaches to being in company with someone with memory loss. From music to food, from painting to storytelling, she invites family members to move past resistance (and understandable grieving) to open themselves to a world of connection through creativity."

Anne Basting
Professor of Theatre, University of Wisconsin–Milwaukee
President, TimeSlips Creative Storytelling

"Deborah uses her experience as a caregiver and years of her own research to create a fun and imaginative guide for caregivers that draws on progress in the arts, physical exercise, and mental stimulation. At its root is the premise that life can still be rich with feeling and meaning even when living with dementia."

Jeffrey M. Burns, MD
Codirector of the University of Kansas Alzheimer's Disease Center

"This uplifting book is really a 'can-do guide' that gives you permission to relax and allow a bit of room for the creative process. The author has a gift for bringing light and love to her writing without minimizing the realities of dementia and caregiving. Deborah understands from a firsthand perspective that a care partner has plenty of duties already, so this book doesn't give the reader the sense that 'there is yet more to add to my to-do list.' Instead, the book is about the infinite possibilities and opportunities to connect, create, and imagine together."

Carmen Mendieta, MPA
Brookdale National Group Respite Program

"Deborah's hopeful spirit comes dancing through in every chapter, with so many wonderful projects and innovators as her partner. All I can say is this: listen to her."

Michelle Niedens, LSCSW
Director of Education, Programs and Public Policy
Alzheimer's Association, Heart of America Chapter

"This book shares stories of compassion and understanding. I found new ways to focus on ensuring quality of life at any level of cognition. It is a must read if you work in elder care settings."

Alisa Tagg, BA, ACC/EDU, AC-BC, CDP
President, National Association of Activity Professionals

"Encouraging, new suggestions for merging caregivers' activities with their loved one's realities of living with dementia."

Leisa Easom, PhD, RN
Executive Director, Pope Eminent Scholar
Rosalynn Carter Institute for Caregiving
Georgia Southwestern State University

"This book inspires people to be creatively engaged. There are many moments to interact play-FULL-y."

Jolene Brackey
Author of *Creating Moments of Joy*

"*Connecting in the Land of Dementia* allows the opportunity to see, in one comprehensive space, the numerous activities and opportunities individuals can have with their loved ones through the course of their dementia. Deborah Shouse and the experts she calls upon provide concrete steps to ensure individuals living with dementia and their caregivers will remain able to live a meaningful life."

Molly Fogel, LCSW
Director of Educational and Social Services,
Alzheimer's Foundation of America

"The opportunity to connect through music, dancing, poetry, and more can lift the hopes of all who want to maintain relationships with those they love late into dementia."

Alicia Ann Clair, PhD
Music Therapist-Board Certified
Professor Emeritus, The University of Kansas, Lawrence

Connecting
in the Land *of*
Dementia

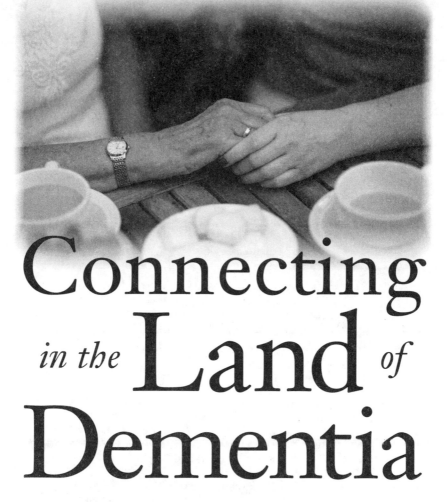

Connecting *in the* Land *of* Dementia

Creative Activities to Explore Together

DEBORAH SHOUSE

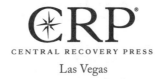

CENTRAL RECOVERY PRESS

Las Vegas

Central Recovery Press (CRP) is committed to publishing exceptional materials addressing addiction treatment, recovery, and behavioral healthcare topics.

For more information, visit www.centralrecoverypress.com.

Publisher: Central Recovery Press
             3321 N. Buffalo Drive
             Las Vegas, NV 89129

21 20 19 18 17 16   1 2 3 4 5

Library of Congress Cataloging-in-Publication Data
Names: Shouse, Deborah, 1949– author.
Title: Connecting in the land of dementia : creative activities to explore
   together / Deborah Shouse.
Description: Las Vegas : Central Recovery Press, [2016]
Identifiers: LCCN 2016019211 (print) | LCCN 2016026281 (ebook) | ISBN
   9781942094241 (paperback) | ISBN 9781942094258 ()
Subjects: LCSH: Alzheimer's disease--Patients--Care. | Alzheimer's
   disease--Patients--Family relationships. | Caregivers. | BISAC: HEALTH &
   FITNESS / Diseases / Alzheimer's & Dementia. | FAMILY & RELATIONSHIPS /
   Eldercare. | MEDICAL / Caregiving. | FAMILY & RELATIONSHIPS / Activities.
Classification: LCC RC523.2 .S5395 2016 (print) | LCC RC523.2 (ebook) | DDC
   616.8/31--dc23
LC record available at https://lccn.loc.gov/2016019211

Photo of Deborah Shouse by Jane Rogers. Used with permission.

Cover design, interior design, and layout by Deb Tremper, Six Penny Graphics.

This book is dedicated to my parents, Frances and Paul Barnett, and to my partner Ron's parents, Mollie and Frank Zoglin. These wonderful people offered us their support, ideas, and guidance, plus a little home cooking and the occasional joke. They showed us the true meaning of love and creativity in the land of dementia. We miss them, yet they live on in our hearts and in the pages of this book.

TABLE OF CONTENTS

How My Desire for Connection Guided Me through the Land of Dementia

For several years, I'd wanted to write about the creative possibilities inherent in being a care partner for someone living with dementia. But I didn't know how to start. The documentary film *Alive Inside* pointed the way. When I watched this powerful movie about music transforming the lives of those living with dementia, I knew I wanted to write about this subject.

I contacted a national magazine and suggested an article. The editor asked, "How else are people communicating with those living with memory loss?" As I researched the question, I discovered a whole new world: Across the globe, writers, painters, musicians, gardeners, dancers, expressive therapists, and other innovators were using the arts, creativity, and imagination as connecting points, tapping into the spirit that thrives in those living with dementia. I was intrigued, and I knew family and professional care partners would also be intrigued and benefit from their ideas.

As my partner Ron and I traveled the world, orchestrating workshops and performing dramatized stories from my book, *Love in the Land of Dementia: Finding Hope in the Caregiver's Journey*, we were inspired by the hundreds of family and professional care partners we met. From Ireland to New Zealand, from Canada to Chile, we all burned with a common passion: to stay deeply connected with those who were living with dementia. And we were not alone. According to the World Alzheimer's Report, by the year 2030, 74.7 million people worldwide will be living with dementia. At this writing, there is no cure. But that doesn't mean there's no hope. The experts I interviewed offer many ways for care partners to stay connected and creative.

This book presents imaginative activities that help you stay linked throughout the dementia journey. These ideas honor the creative spirit, reminding us we can all make a difference, one painting, one song, one smile, one shared experience at a time.

SECTION I
Creativity and Imagination Matter

CHAPTER ONE

Discover the Wonders in the Dementia Jungle

Look beyond the Thorns

Sneak Previews

Outsmart Personal Resistance

Get Started

Look beyond the Thorns

"All great changes are preceded by chaos." —Deepak Chopra

"Excuse me Deborah, but you may not want to touch these trees," Pablo, our guide, gently suggested.

We were slogging down a narrow, muddy, jungle path in the Ecuadorian rainforest, and I had grabbed onto a branch to steady myself. I glanced at the branch; my hand was surrounded by serious-looking black thorns. I wobbled as I plunged my hand into my pocket.

"Those thorns are poisonous," Pablo said. "They can temporarily paralyze you. But you recover."

I tucked my hand into my shirtsleeve so I wouldn't be tempted to latch onto another tree. I wondered what I was doing, trekking around in such a chaotic and unknown environment, among paralyzing thorns, biting ants, and venomous snakes. Then I looked up at the towering canopy of lush leaves. I noticed a wild orchid shyly clinging to the thorn tree. Pablo pointed to the hollow in a nearby tree trunk, and I saw a baby night monkey peeking out, its large brown eyes inquisitive as a child's. A scarlet macaw squawked by and a line of leaf cutter ants marched past my hiking boots, each boldly toting greenery twice its size. The poison thorns seemed a small price to pay for such an extraordinarily rich and vibrant experience.

The journey through dementia can be similar. My partner, Ron, and I trekked through the dementia jungle with three of our four parents. We tried hard to keep our parents stimulated and engaged. We had our thorny moments and we had deep moments of wonder. We learned the power of creativity and imagination.

We also learned that even when people can no longer drive to the grocery store or remember their grandchildren's names, their lives can still be rich. In fact, because their reactions are sometimes less filtered and more honest, their creative powers are often heightened.

Creative Projects Jazz Up the Day and Light Up the Spirit

Too often, people living with dementia are entertained instead of engaged. Their lifelong activities are stripped away, and they have little to do. Research shows that artistic and imaginative activities reduce the need for psychotropic medications. With such engagement, people's sense of well-being and purpose improves. Agitation and depression can diminish. Doing activities together increases social interactions, builds positive energy, and adds a sense of discovery to the day.

These creative activities benefit family and professional care partners as well. According to Sarah Zoutewelle-Morris, author of *Chocolate Rain: 100 Ideas for a Creative Approach to Activities in Dementia Care*, participating in projects allows a mutual exchange: You give to the person living with dementia, and she gives to you. Working or playing together lowers stress and can bring an increased sense of peace.

> Research shows that artistic and imaginative activities reduce the need for psychotropic medications.

"The creative approach is a sincere belief in people's potential, celebrating who they are, respecting them, and supporting their autonomy," says Sarah. "Anything can be a meaningful activity. It's all about helping people express themselves."

The ideas and activities in this book will add joy and substance to your time with people who are living with dementia. As a bonus, these exercises are also a boost for you. Increasingly, studies show that painting, drawing, and other arts and crafts reduce the risk of cognitive impairment. Additional activities such as music, movement, gardening, and social interactions strengthen the body, brain, and spirit.

Increasingly, studies show that painting, drawing, and other arts and crafts reduce the risk of cognitive impairment. Additional activities such as music, movement, gardening, and social interactions strengthen the body, brain, and spirit.

Sneak Previews

"Creativity is contagious, pass it on." —Albert Einstein

For years, I've been interviewing people who use creativity, imagination, and expressive therapies to connect with people living with dementia. These experts helped me translate their groundbreaking ideas into simple projects that family and professional care partners can use.

Here are a few sneak previews of the transformative benefits:

As usual, Henry is slumped silently in his wheelchair, eyes closed, hands listless in his lap. Dan Cohen puts the headphones on Henry and turns on the MP3 player, which is programmed with Henry's favorite tunes from the 1940s. When the music starts, Henry suddenly raises his head and opens his eyes. He smiles, snaps his fingers, and taps his feet, echoing his old dance steps. Such responses to music fueled the international Music and Memory movement. Today, thousands of people living with dementia are waking up their creative spirits through music.

•—•

Nan often spent long hours playing solitaire with a well-worn deck of cards. But when her confusion increased, her dexterity diminished, and her eyesight dimmed, she could no longer handle the deck, and her daughter sadly put away the cards. Then her daughter bought a computer tablet boasting a touch screen. She showed her mother how to play solitaire by simply touching the desired card and moving it, on the screen, to the proper pile. Now they both enjoy huddling together and discussing strategies. The card game has become an important part of their weekly visit.

●—●

At first, Gary Glazner thinks everyone in the dayroom is asleep. The memory care residents are silently slumped in chairs and wheelchairs. But Gary is determined to share the verses he brought.

"I shot an arrow into the air," he reads.

"And it came down, I know not where," a man in a wheelchair replies. Even though his head is bowed and his eyes are closed, the familiar poem resonates with him.

Experiences like this were the catalyst for Gary Glazner's Poetry Project, a global outreach that encourages communicating through poetry.

●—●

For some people, the spark comes through music; others are moved by storytelling, theater, dance, movement, cooking, technology, art, or gardening. This book shows you simple ways to use these art forms to relate to people who are living with dementia.

Today, thousands of people living with dementia are waking up their creative spirits through music.

Outsmart Personal Resistance

"You need chaos in your soul to give birth
to a dancing star." —Friedrich Nietzsche

The demands on your time are legion. Your stresses are mountains, and your periods of calm and solitude are as rare as snow leopards. When people encourage you to try various activities to connect with a person living with dementia, you may think, *Why bother? She won't remember anyway. She won't like it or won't agree to participate. Besides, I don't have time, I'm worn out, and I'm not creative.*

Yet, there are many reasons to pursue creative connections. The experts I interviewed for this book believe imaginative activities boost energy and increase the ways to stay connected and stimulated. These interactions can also add purpose to your lives.

"Meaningful activities have to be as big a priority
as medicine, bathing, and meal times."

Marie Marley, PhD, former care partner and coauthor (with neurologist Daniel C. Potts, MD, FAAN) of *Finding Joy in Alzheimer's: New Hope for Caregivers,* has experienced going beyond resistance. Marie's beloved partner Ed was a devotee of classical music. When he developed dementia, friends suggested Marie and Ed listen to symphonic recordings together. But that sounded boring to Marie, and for weeks she resisted the recommendation. Then one day, when conversation with Ed wasn't working, she put on some Mozart. Ed instantly began moving with the music.

Knowing how Ed loved a flamboyant conductor, Marie waved her arms, tossed her head, and jumped up and down, urging the invisible orchestra to play its heart out. Ed was thrilled. Afterward he told her, "That was really beautiful."

"Once I overcame my resistance, I intuitively knew I should emulate a conductor." Marie says. "Listening to music became a meaningful way to spend time together."

Later, Marie hired a violinist who arrived, suited up in a tuxedo, to play a special concert for Ed.

"Ed loved the experience," Marie says. "I knew he wouldn't remember it, but you have to live in the moment. Research shows that even if people don't remember, their joy and happiness can linger on."

Marie learned to encourage Ed to try new things and was surprised when he enjoyed pursuits he would never have considered in earlier life. She also learned to try something different if an idea didn't seem to be working.

"When you find activities you like, it's great for both of you," Marie says.

Author Mara Botonis agrees: "Meaningful activities have to be as big a priority as medicine, bathing, and meal times."

Get Started

"The project might not look like it is going as planned, but to your partner it may feel simply marvelous!" —Carmen Mendieta

If you want to feel more connected to someone who's living with dementia, if you want to add meaning to daily life and work, if you want a dash of inspiration and a long cool drink of hope, then you'll enjoy exploring this book.

The experts I interviewed graciously shared real-life examples. I have changed the names of those living with dementia to protect their privacy. Also, to avoid excess wordiness, I will often refer to people living with dementia as "your partner." Whether you are a family member, friend, or a healthcare professional, you'll appreciate partnering for these creative projects and activities.

I've divided the book into topics. Each segment reveals the benefits and offers the reader succinct how-tos in the form of **Creative Sparks**. These activities are participatory and adaptable for people of varying physical and mental abilities. You can enjoy them one-on-one or in a group, either at home or in a care community setting. Some of these ideas may seem easy, while others may appear more challenging. I encourage you to sample them all.

CHAPTER TWO

Make the Most of This Book

Take a New Look at the Yellow Crayon

Embrace the Why, How, and Wow

Take a New Look at the Yellow Crayon

"To live a creative life, we must lose our fear of being wrong." —Joseph Chilton Pierce

Before he leaves for his outing, my father beckons me out onto the ramshackle porch of the rental cottage. He solemnly hands me a tablet of thick, white artist's paper and a pristine box of twenty-four crayons.

"I want you to get your mother interested in art again," he says. "I believe she can still draw and paint, but she resists when I mention it. You're the only one who can help her."

My parents, my brother's family, and my two daughters and I are on a family trip to Hot Springs, Arkansas. Mom has been struggling with forgetfulness and odd behaviors (or rather, Dad has been struggling with her forgetfulness and odd behaviors) for a couple of years. As long as Mom is near Dad, she seems happy enough, paddling around in the swimming pool, being near her young grandchildren, and reminiscing about her earlier life. But when Dad takes even a short break, Mom's mouth tightens and her eyes search wildly. "Where is . . . ?" she asks, over and over again, twisting her hands.

Today, my father is joining my brother and the children for boating and tubing. Since Mom doesn't like such heat and noise, I volunteer to spend the day with her.

I nod gravely when my father hands me the "art supplies." I seriously believe I, Super Daughter and Muse, can fulfill my father's request to reunite my mother and her passion for art.

I haven't yet accepted Mom for who she is now. I'm still grieving the loss of the mom I've always known, and I earnestly believe that the best possible idea is to return her to the artist, mother, wife, and grandmother she used to be.

That afternoon, shortly after Dad leaves, I lure Mom to the small Formica kitchen table with coffee and chocolate chip cookies.

"Where is . . . ?" Mom asks, knotting together her fingers.

"He's out with Dan and the kids. They're going boating," I tell her. "He won't be gone too long."

Mom stares at me accusingly.

"Where is Paul?" she says, her voice wobbly.

"He's with the kids. He'll be back soon."

I hand her a sheet of paper and take one for myself. I spread the crayons out and say, "Let's draw."

"Why?" she says.

"Because it's fun," I say, touching her hand and looking into her eyes, just as I imagine a muse might do. "Because you enjoy making art. You're good at it."

After I left home for college, sketching and painting became Mom's creative mainstays. She produced hundreds of paintings, often bringing to life old photographs that captured a snippet of family history: Dad's father appearing wickedly self-confident in a game of poker; her own mother, before she immigrated to America, as a shy young woman with an upswept Gibson girl hairdo; her grandchildren dancing around my den in a mad-cap talent show. But she hasn't touched a brush or pencil in several years, and Dad has mourned mightily over her abandoning this passion.

"Where is . . . ?" Mom asks.

"Let's make a picture for Dad," I say. "He'll be thrilled."

I hand Mom a yellow crayon and I pick up a purple one. I draw a series of squiggling lines. I add in a green, then a blue. I envision Dad's beaming face when Mom hands him her sketch of yellow roses. I imagine his warm hug and his grateful, whispered words, "Thanks, Debbie. I knew you could do it. I feel like your mother's come home."

My wild, colorful lines fill the page. Finally, I glance up, ready to admire Mom's work. But all I see is a blinding sheet of yellow. She has scrubbed the yellow crayon across the page. No flowers, no independent lines, no blending of colors. I bite my lip, tasting bitter failure, and imagining the look of despair on my father's face.

That was before I had learned to let go of Mom as a representational artist and embrace her mellow yellow creation. That was before I accepted the challenge of journeying to my mom's current world instead of struggling unsuccessfully to drag her back into mine. I finally did let go and embraced my mom as she was. Mom learned to laugh at her forgetfulness; she learned to communicate with smiles and gestures; she learned the art of living in the moment. And I learned along with her.

Today, if I could once again sit beside her and color, I would simply enjoy the process and not set myself up as a failed Super Muse. I might just say, "I love the brightness of that color," and not yearn for a bouquet of roses that would prove Mom was the same as ever.

I might see if she and I could draw something together. We'd take turns making lines on the paper, sketching out a nonverbal dialogue. I'd play some of her favorite songs while we drew, and we'd sing along. I might include some soothing lavender tea, accompanied by decadent chocolate chip cookies. Whatever we did together, I would cherish that shared time.

Embrace the Why, How, and Wow

"People with dementia are my best teachers, constantly offering me insights and giving me new ways of seeing, hearing, and experiencing things." —Teepa Snow

Daily visits and interactions are a vital part of care partnering. "Our responsibility is to connect with and bring people out," says Cameron Camp, PhD, coauthor of *A Different Visit*. "Activities allow us to rediscover the person who may be hiding behind his or her deficit."

A good activity should be easy, mutually pleasurable, appropriate for ability, age, and gender, imbued with some meaning, and have no deadline and no pressure. You don't need any special artistic talent to facilitate and enjoy these ideas. Here are some ways to get started.

"Activities allow us to rediscover the person who may be hiding behind his or her deficit."

Ask Others to Join You

> "Our basic instincts include discovery and invention, and thus creativity. These abilities are hard-wired, and people living with dementia can still draw on these skills."

Though John Zeisel has a doctorate in sociology from Columbia University and has studied and taught in prestigious colleges and universities, he says several of his most significant teachers were persons living with dementia. Until he was in his forties, John hadn't known many people living with Alzheimer's. He worked in environmental design, and an opportunity to redesign a memory care facility changed both his career path and his life. He grew fascinated by the openness, sensitivity, and creativity of those living with memory loss and began studying neuroscience.

"Our basic instincts include discovery and invention, and thus creativity," John says. "These abilities are hard-wired, and people living with dementia can still draw on these skills. They are often exceptionally perceptive, increasingly creative, and have high emotional intelligence. It's our job to uncover and embrace their abilities so they maintain dignity, independence, and self-respect."

Many care partners struggle through a period of grief, helplessness, and anger when a loved one receives a dementia diagnosis. But if care partners and families can move from despair into hopefulness, they can access their natural curiosity. Hope, to John, means knowing that we can make a difference in the person's life. With hope, we all become creative and wonder, *What is going on and how can I make a difference?*

John, the author of *I'm Still Here: A New Philosophy of Alzheimer's Care*, often facilitates conversations about the "gifts" in the care partnering experience. He suggests a family, along with significant friends, get together and ask the person living with dementia, "How can I make a difference for you? What can I do to make things a little bit better?"

Once all have responded to this request, they can all then discuss, "How can we support and help each other as a group?" John calls this a Circle of Hope.

"Every family member and friend can make a difference in the life of the person living with dementia," John says.

Focus on Personal Preferences

Focusing on your partner's passions helps you select and adapt meaningful projects. Jackie Pinkowitz is a pioneer in the international Person-Centered Living movement (PCL), which sees people as whole, regardless of disabilities, including dementia. According to PCL, all people with disabilities are entitled to choice, privacy, respect, and autonomy. Any assistance they need should be centered on their personal preferences and values.

> Focusing on your partner's passions helps you select and adapt meaningful projects.

"Ultimately, this philosophy means being kind and sensitive and honoring people's right to make their own choices," Jackie says. "With this attitude of openness, you can help people live fully with dementia, enriching their lives with meaning, community engagement, and social relationships."

Issue the Invitation

As an artist, Sarah Zoutewelle-Morris was excited about her new job as an activities director in the Netherlands. Previously, she had been part of a performing troupe that staged artistic events in healthcare institutions. She was used to instantly connecting and making people smile. But in the care setting, when she took out her art supplies and invited people to join, the residents backed away, saying, "That's for kids," or "I don't want to do that."

"I learned I couldn't confront people with creativity too soon," she says. "I couldn't go in as the artist; I had to figure out ways to invite people into a project."

In South Dakota, Ari Albright, an artist in residence in a dementia unit, has had similar experiences.

"If I said, 'Hey, want to make art?' people shied away, saying, 'I can't draw, I can't paint. I don't know what to do,'" Ari says.

But if Ari asked, "Do you have a moment to help me?" or "Would you give me a hand?" people were interested in assisting.

"It's all about issuing the right kind of invitation," Ari says.

Offer Choices and Encourage Ideas

Whenever possible offer two or three choices. "Shall we start with the blue, red, or green paint?" "Shall we listen to 'Blue Moon' or 'Fly Me to the Moon'?"

Slow down and allow time for your partner to process. "Before you help, let the person tussle with the task a bit," Ari suggests.

Encourage whatever ideas come up.

"The least intrusive way to communicate is by signaling someone with a gesture or expression," Ari says. "When you need to speak, gently repeat words as often as necessary. Or you can show by example, placing the person's hand over your hand as you draw, paint, or put something together."

Give people notice as you're winding down the project. Thank them for their help and offer a low-key transition, such as "I'm putting away these materials now. It's time to clean up the table and get ready for dinner. Will you join me?"

Say Yes and Create a Failure-Free Zone

"That's salad dressing, not milk. Don't drink that."

"No, we're not going to see Sissy today; we're seeing her next month."

"Watch out for that pen; you're getting ink all over your shirt."

What if you were constantly being told no and assured you were mistaken, clumsy, or wrong? Care partners have the difficult balancing act of keeping people safe while nurturing their self-esteem and independence.

> With activities, you can invite unfettered self-expression by suspending judgment and saying yes to ideas.

Imagine knowing what you want to do and not being able to communicate your wishes. For example, Emily wants to step outside to look at the roses, but the words are stuck in her throat. So she walks down the hall to the outside door. A woman steps into her path. The woman's smile is too big, and her voice is too high.

"Where are you going?" she asks.

Emily gestures toward the door but the woman shakes her head.

"No, you can't go home," she says. "But you can go to Bingo. Come back this way with me."

The woman doesn't understand, but Emily cannot explain herself. "The roses," Emily wants to tell her, "I want to smell and touch them. They're just like the ones I used to grow at home."

Teepa Snow, an occupational therapist who teaches dementia care across the nation, understands how frustrated Emily is feeling. For years, she has worked with people who have trouble using words to communicate. She knows that the tone of voice matters and authenticity is key.

"I imagine how I would feel if I couldn't express my needs and someone was telling me, 'No, no, no,'" Teepa says.

With activities, you can invite unfettered self-expression by suspending judgment and saying yes to ideas. This removes the risk of embarrassment, reduces the fear of making a mistake, and helps your partner feel creative, capable, and loved.

Redefine Being Helpful

Teepa has also seen well-meaning caregivers be too helpful. That's what happened to George.

George loves jigsaw puzzles, but no matter how hard he tries, the pieces simply won't fit together.

"Don't worry, Dad," says that nice woman who takes care of him. "I'll help you."

She quickly fits a whole section together. George knew he was getting dumber, and this proves it. Why should he even bother to do another puzzle? He'd like to have just a little assistance, but the words won't fit together so he can let that nice woman know.

"We need to redefine what it means to be helpful," Teepa says. "Instead of doing something for people, we can offer choices. This increases their sense of independence and control."

If someone is struggling to find a missing puzzle piece, put your hand under hers and guide her to two pieces, then together experiment to see which one will fit. By collaborating, you're supporting and empowering the person living with dementia.

Go with the Flow

Perhaps you've experienced something like this: You've set up a wonderful tea time, complete with your mom's favorite cucumber sandwiches, English breakfast tea, a clip from one of her favorite British comedies, and some photos from a long ago trip to the United Kingdom. Everything is ready to go, except your mom, who is gazing out the window at a starling and worrying a hole in her favorite red cardigan.

After you have a moment of disappointment, go with the flow and tailor the activity to her mood.

If she's staring out the window, take her outside, if possible. Or find nature photos and sounds and experience those together. If she's rocking back and forth in her chair, or repeating a folding motion, support her rhythmic movements with music or light tapping.

Make a List of Likes

Even for the most dedicated, being a care partner is not easy. Teepa Snow recommends making a list of the things you like about the person with dementia.

You might write, "I like the way he laughs." That will direct you to watch for humorous moments. "I like her curiosity." You can search out new projects to stimulate both of you. "I like the way he appreciates nature." You'll explore ways to be outside and experiment with ways to bring nature indoors.

When challenges arise in your interactions, this list reminds you to focus on the qualities you most appreciate.

Creative Sparks

★ Choose a quiet space relatively free of distractions. Select a time of day when you and your partner both have lively energy.

★ Choose a project you'd both enjoy and ready your supplies.

★ Issue the invitation and set the psychological stage for a failure-free activity.

★ Tap into your own spirit of playfulness. Take risks and try new things. Celebrate whatever happens, whether it's an amazing watercolor drawing or yellow marks on plain white paper.

★ Allow the project to unfold at its own pace, offering support as necessary and encouragement along the way.

★ Know when to take a break. If you don't have energy to be curious, if you're exhausted, take a break and come back to the activity later. Otherwise you'll feel frustrated.

★ If the project doesn't go as planned, don't worry. Go with the flow, praise the effort, and acknowledge the skill. Try again another day, choose another project, or try a variation of the activity.

★ Give notice when you're winding down and offer an easy transition into whatever is next.

★ Thank the person for being part of this activity with you.

SECTION II

Meaningful Projects for People Living with Dementia and Their Care Partners

CHAPTER THREE

Strengthen Communications through Creativity

Explore New Ways of Connecting

Join the Dementia Revolution

Reinvent Favorite Hobbies

Use Playfulness to Jump-Start Conversations

Say Yes to Improv

Spice Up Communications

Discover the Creativity at the End of the Rainbow

Explore New Ways of Connecting

"Where words no longer brought us together, something richer did . . . a universal expression, a deeper knowing . . . a place where the resilient human spirit, against all odds, rises to meet itself and seek another." —Laura Beck

Laura Beck knows firsthand the wonders of creativity and dementia. Laura, who is the Learning and Development Guide at The Eden Alternative, began her informal studies on dementia

when she was in her early thirties. Her father was living in a
Texas nursing home that was practicing The Eden Alternative.
This philosophy, developed by Jude and Bill Thomas, MD, helps
families and care professionals create quality of life through
compassionate care partnerships that put the person first.

Laura's dad had been a competitive ballroom dancer, and
he resonated with music. Though he'd lost his speech, he could
express himself verbally through jazz scat (rhythmic syllables, such
as "be-dop-a-do-bop.")

One evening, Laura went to visit him. She heard him singing
and followed his voice to his room. He was lying in bed, his thick
white hair wildly tousled, his eyes wide, and his voice loud, primal,
and totally alive. To Laura, he looked like a shaman or warrior.
His intense, primitive sounds startled her and for a moment, she
felt so overwhelmed, she stepped out of the room.

That could be me, she thought, steadying herself against the
doorframe and taking a deep breath. Once she acknowledged her
feelings, she felt stronger. She walked back into the room and sat
beside her father, took his hand, and stared into his hazel eyes.
Each time he chanted something, she offered affirmations, saying,
"Yes, I hear you." Then she noticed he was having more fun than
she was. She began responding to his chants, repeating them in
a call and response. For twenty minutes, her dad called out with
fiery syllables, and his daughter echoed him.

"Those were the most connected moments I ever had with him,"
Laura says. "For me, that was a template for being creative in a
relationship. My father brought me into the present and invited
me to play."

That experience helped Laura understand in a new way what it
meant to be a care partner.

"Every moment, we're both recipient and giver," she says.

> "Until we address our own issues with
> dementia and aging, we cannot step into an
> open and expressive care partnership."

"During the dementia journey, creativity makes space for spontaneity and possibility," she says. "Anytime we can listen to the wisdom of people living with dementia and give them voice and audience, we can learn something profound and powerful."

She saw her father's innate wisdom and realized the importance of noticing and dealing with her own fears.

"Until we address our own issues with dementia and aging, we cannot step into an open and expressive care partnership," Laura says.

In the pages ahead, you'll find ways to add expressiveness, comfort, playfulness, and depth into your everyday conversations.

Join the Dementia Revolution

"What if we treated people who were living with dementia like we treated children who were living with Down syndrome? What if we said Alzheimer's syndrome instead of Alzheimer's disease?" —Cameron Camp, PhD

Sandra's hands are sweating as she walks into the building. She knows her father needs memory care, yet she feels sad, guilty, and worried about him living in a facility. As she waits to meet with the marketing person, a nicely dressed older gentleman approaches and introduces himself. "I'll be taking you on a tour of the community," Franklin says.

Sandra almost rolls her eyes at the word "community." Just jargon to help the families feel more at ease, she figures. She follows him into the memory care unit, expecting to be assaulted by offensive smells and stagnating elders. Instead, she is greeted by vibrant art, fresh flowers, and a lively mixture of people clustered around a piano, singing along. Franklin explains the various programs, showing her the cooking counter in the spacious dining area, where community members and kitchen staff are chopping red and yellow peppers for a Mexican lunch. After a tour of the library, he shows her a typical resident bedroom, then invites her into another bedroom filled with a variety of plants.

"This is my room," Franklin says. "I'm a gardener, as you can see."

Sandra tries to mask her surprise. She had no idea that Franklin was living with dementia. And she had no idea that her father could keep on gardening once he moved into a home.

> "We are constantly asking ourselves, 'What would people living with dementia want to do if they didn't have a memory impairment?' and 'How can we help them do that?'"

Cameron Camp, PhD, has worked with Franklin's care home, using Montessori and other person-centered principles. Cameron is the author of *Montessori-Based Activities for Persons with Dementia, Volumes 1 and 2.* He's an international leader in using Montessori principles to help people living with dementia keep engaged and connected. Maria Montessori originally designed her program to help disadvantaged children who struggled with learning and other disabilities. One of her precepts is, "Help me to help myself." As Cameron trains care partners all over the world, he emphasizes the values of respect, dignity, and equality.

Cameron says, "We are constantly asking ourselves, 'What would people living with dementia want to do if they didn't have a memory impairment?' and 'How can we help them do that?'"

Leading with Reading

That kind of thinking led Cameron and his team at the Center for Applied Research in Dementia to develop the Reading Roundtable®. Franklin facilitates a group discussion, attended by people with all levels of dementia, including the later stages. Topics range from the invention of basketball, to the life of Leonardo da Vinci, to the history of the chocolate chip cookie. Each participant receives an eight-inch by ten-inch booklet with a colorful cover and large, bold print on each page. Franklin begins by reading the first page, which describes the wonderful aroma of fresh-baked chocolate chip cookies.

> "According to our research, when persons with early to moderate dementia lead reading and discussion groups, attendees are happier and more constructively engaged than they are when staff leads the group."

Franklin asks the group, "Who baked cookies in your growing up household?"

One woman says, "My mother."

Another says, "I did."

Then he goes around the table, asking the next person to read a page, assisting anyone who needs help. Along the way, he continues to ask questions, and they get into interesting conversations.

"According to our research, when persons with early to moderate dementia lead reading and discussion groups, attendees are happier and more constructively engaged than they are when staff leads the group," Cameron says.

Treat People as We Wish to be Treated

> Instead of focusing on, 'Look what they *can't do*,' we celebrate, 'Look what they *can do* with assistance.'

"We simply try to treat people living with dementia as we wish to be treated," he says. "We follow Montessori's guidelines, trying to help people regain control of their lives."

Montessori said, "Everything you do for me, you take away from me." To keep this from happening, Cameron and his team work with families and facilities to create an environment where everyone enjoys responsibilities, purpose, and meaningful social roles. Examples include empowering people living in care settings (or at home) to greet new people, memorializing those who pass away, visiting friends who are in the hospital, and deciding what kinds of outings they want to experience.

> "We are attempting to revolutionize the way we treat and think about dementia."

Cameron encourages intergenerational work. He creates workstations, where people living with dementia can mentor young children, showing them how to use work tools, bake a cake, hang up clothes, make model boats, knit, and more.

He supports families in creating cognitive ramps. "Similar to physical ramps for people who are in wheelchairs, cognitive ramps help people overcome challenges so they more fully participate.

Instead of focusing on, 'Look what they *can't do*,' we celebrate, 'Look what they *can do* with assistance.'"

What they can do is legion. Take the open mic comedy club created and staffed by people living with dementia. They send invitations to family and friends. They select and print the jokes, and they find a singer to entertain between acts. The singer types the lyrics to all the songs he knows and prints them. When guests arrive, two gentlemen who are wearing tuxedos guide them to their tables. A waitress asks, "Tea, lemonade, red wine, or white wine?"

"Tea," a guest might answer.

The waitress places a brown square beside him. "Please don't move that or I won't know what kind of drink to pour," she explains. She knows the brown square equals ice tea; the red square equals red wine. This Montessori matching exercise allows her to fill the social role of the server and outshine the memory issues. To set the tables, she consults a template—a drawing on a placemat that outlines fork, spoon, knife, glass, napkin, and plate.

"We are attempting to revolutionize the way we treat and think about dementia," Cameron says. "People want to live well with dementia, just as they want to live well with diabetes and cancer."

Creative Sparks

★ Notice your partner's interests and abilities.

★ Build on strengths by developing "cognitive ramps," which can help your partner stay active and engaged and living his best life.

★ Incorporate Montessori principles into your activities. These include using materials you can hold and

manipulate, offering choices, and demonstrating the
activity first.

★ Use matching principles and templates to expand and
enhance activities.

Reinvent Favorite Hobbies

"Let the things you love be your escape." —Anonymous

"My mom loves gardening, but with her memory loss she just
can't work outside anymore."

During her career as an executive in the senior living industry,
Mara Botonis often heard this kind of lament from family
members. When her own beloved grandfather was diagnosed with
dementia, she was determined that he would continue to enjoy his
lifelong passions, which included golf, playing cards, and fishing.

"I wanted Grandfather to have the best possible
experience every day, so I learned to put
laughing ahead of laundry and dishes."

Mara, author of *When Caring Takes Courage: A Compassionate,
Interactive Guide for Alzheimer's and Dementia Caregivers*,
understood the care partner's tendency to let creative time slide
in favor of vital practical matters, such as assisting with dressing,
feeding, and bathing.

"I wanted Grandfather to have the best possible experience every day, so I learned to put laughing ahead of laundry and dishes," she says. "So what if we use throw-away paper plates?"

Here are some ways Mara successfully kept her grandfather involved in his passions. For a time, he walked the golf course and played with empathetic friends. When he could no longer play, he liked being driven around the course, enjoying the scent of freshly mown grass, the vistas of rolling green lawns, and the thwack of a well-hit ball. At home, the family set up an indoor putting green and watched golf tournaments on television with him.

Family gin rummy sessions were another of her grandfather's favorites. When he could no longer track the game, Mara asked herself, "What is important about these family competitions?" She realized the game was a catalyst for reminiscing, laughing, and eating their ritual potato chips and dip. Even when Grandfather couldn't play, he still liked sorting the cards by suits and sitting around the card table with his family.

Mara helped Grandfather stay involved in fishing by taking him out on a boat when he could no longer navigate on his own. On other days, they'd walk by the shore, stopping to chat with fishermen, smelling the salty breeze, and watching the sea birds. Back home, Mara encouraged him to organize a tackle box, by sorting and arranging the hook-less lures.

To adapt your own projects, ask yourself: What is most important about the activity? For example, for gardeners, is it the feel of their hands in the soil? Is it producing flowers or harvesting vegetables? Having something to take care of? For those who like quilting, is it the finished product or making the squares? Is it the companionship with other quilters? Or the feel of the fabric? With that information, you can break down the components of the activities and see which are doable and pleasing.

Creative Sparks

★ Discuss which hobbies and rituals are most important to your partner.

★ List the components of the experience and learn which parts your partner most enjoys.

★ Adapt the experience as needed to your partner's changing interests.

Use Playfulness to Jump-Start Conversations

"Love, the essence of love, manifests itself through playfulness."—Réné Gaudette

For days, Albert sat in front of the television, stony-faced, unmoving. His wife Grace tried to pry him loose by asking, "Want to go for a walk?" But Albert sat silent, eventually mumbling, "No." Then Grace talked to Erin Bonitto, a Minnesota-based dementia communication coach. Afterward, instead of hovering meekly in front of the television waiting for her husband to answer her, Grace turned off the program, sat beside Albert, and glanced all around the room.

"Albert," she said, "You're the best looking man in the room."

Albert chuckled.

"We should stretch our legs," Grace said. "Come with me, I have something to show you."

Albert stood and went with Grace.

"It's not so much what you say," Erin says. "You're trying to create a spark and connection between you." As founder and lead coach in Gemini Consulting, Life Enrichment Systems for Dementia, Erin has years of experience working with care partners in home and healthcare settings.

Jazz Up Visits

Nan didn't know what to say when she visited her mom in the memory care community. If she said, "Hi Mom, how are you?" she'd either hear, "Fine," or she'd be bombarded by her mom's list of complaints.

Erin advised Nan to stride in with a big smile and open body language. Instead of a routine question, she might say, "Wow Mom, you look like a million dollars." Or, "Mom, you look so good I think we should go out for a stroll."

> "You're trying to restore creativity and playfulness to your relationship."

Another daughter took Erin's suggestion to a higher level and said to her widowed mother, "Mom, you're so beautiful today, I think we should go find some men."

"I think we should too," her mom answered.

Erin explains, "You're trying to restore creativity and playfulness to your relationship."

Playfulness worked its magic with another family. Whenever Jack wandered into his kitchen with a look of confusion on his face, his wife learned to say something cheerful, such as, "At last. The King has arrived." Then she laughed, and Jack chuckled as well.

"The laughter releases endorphins," Erin says. "Once those endorphins are moving, conversation flows more easily. When you use these techniques, you are both on the exact same plane."

Have Fun and Break Ice

Erin is working with the staff of a memory care home in Minnesota to help their residents more readily interact with each other.

"These residents have a capacity for friendship and joking, but they can't initiate a conversation," Erin explains. "We're coaching the staff on ways to connect by using irreverent ice breakers."

For example, an aide guides Joe to his seat at the dining table. "Harry," the aide says to another man at the same table, "Keep an eye on Joe. He's a real troublemaker." She smiles and both Harry and Joe laugh. They are now connected and talking.

Creative Sparks

★ Think of phrases that will surprise and please your partner, such as:

For a spouse:

★ "Ah . . . it's the lady I've been waiting for!"

★ "You know, I haven't had a single hug today."

★ "Ah, my partner in crime!"

For a parent or grandparent:

★"Well, there's my distinguished dad!"

★"Mom, it's me, your best-looking daughter!"

★ When your conversation becomes rote, add in phrases and gestures that will evoke a smile or laugh.

★ Help your partner communicate with others by offering playful introductions.

Say Yes to Improv

"To succeed, planning alone is insufficient. One must improvise as well." —Isaac Asimov

Karen's mom gazes out the window and notices squirrels jumping from one tree to the next. She has never seen squirrels leap so high, and she assumes they are a different animal.

"Look at those monkeys," her mom says.

"Yes and they're jumping all around," Karen answers, inviting her mom's creativity instead of correcting her. "What shall we do with them?"

"Catch one," her mom answers. "Look at those monkeys."

"Yes and they're flying from branch to branch," Karen says.

"And they're wishing for a banana," her mom says, smiling.

Karen smiles. They are two women, monkeying around, engaging in a stimulating exchange.

Yes, Yes, and Again Yes

Because of her background in improvisational theater, Karen Stobbe of North Carolina, often relies on "Yes, and . . ." a key component of any skit.

"With both improv and caregiving, you learn the basics; then you go with the flow."

"When you say no, you stop the flow of language," Karen says. "'Yes, and . . .' invites imagination and creativity."

Karen got the idea for using improv techniques with her mom when she was suffering through a boring caregivers' workshop. Karen thought, "If I see one more PowerPoint slide showing one more grim brain picture, I'll explode. If only they'd use some improvisation games, they could illustrate the information more clearly."

She had worked as an actor, writer, and improv artist. To keep her sanity during the endless workshop, she began jotting down improvisational ideas that would help caregivers.

"With both improv and caregiving, you learn the basics; then you go with the flow," Karen says. "You can rehearse, but you're only practicing techniques. The performance remains a surprise."

Karen fleshed out her ideas, received a grant, and created a training program that she offers free on her website. The program has also helped Karen enliven her communications with her mom.

The Flow Is Fun

When communicating with a person living with dementia, Karen suggests, "Go with the flow. Don't contradict, argue, or question. As family members, we often hang onto the past and desperately want our loved ones to be 'normal.' They are being normal in their world, and we need to step into that arena."

In improv, as in caregiving, you don't put the other person on the spot. In a skit, if you ask a pointed question, you give unwanted power to the other person. In a care situation, you're asking a question of someone who may struggle with the answer and feel frustrated.

So when Karen takes her mom to their favorite ice cream shop, she doesn't ask, "Do you know where are we right now?" Instead, Karen anchors her mom by saying, "This is a really beautiful ice cream shop. Look at all the flavors and think about what you'd like."

If her mom seems overwhelmed by the rainbow of choices, Karen says, "I'm going to get a scoop of chocolate. You usually like Rocky Road. Is that what you'd like today or do you want to try French Vanilla?"

Back home, Karen understands her mom's worry over making mistakes. So she doesn't say, "Mom, want to sit down and I'll bring you a snack." Karen knows her mom will stand frozen in front of the table, not knowing which place is hers. Instead, Karen walks her mom to the chair and pulls it out for her.

"Here's your chair, Mom," Karen says. "Would you like to sit here or on the couch?"

Allow for Silence

In both improv and caregiving, sometimes you don't know what to do or how to respond. When you feel stuck, you can simply say, "I don't know what to say right now. Let me think." Several minutes of quiet can clear your mind and inspire insights.

Creative Sparks

★ Use improv techniques for more open and creative communication.

★ Encourage conversation by saying, "Yes and . . . ."

★ Try not to correct your partner.

★ Go with the flow. If your mom is confused and believes you are an old friend, allow her the comfort of communicating with that person.

★ Welcome silence. When you don't know what to do, a few moments of silence or deep breathing can restore you.

Spice Up Communications

"We must work intuitively and creatively—
remembering the dementia journey goes beyond
alienation into wonderment." —Karrie Marshall

Once her husband, Colin, is dressed, Angela hands him a postcard that reads, "You are invited to try a brand new breakfast cereal this morning." The previous morning, Colin's invitation promised, "You are invited to watch a new television program with me today. Popcorn included."

"An invitation creates an occasion and adds a bright focus to the day," says Karrie Marshall, author of *Puppetry in Dementia Care*.

"You gain something new to talk about and something different to experience together."

Karrie, a former nurse, lives in Inverness, Scotland, and specializes in creative projects for those living with dementia. Invitation ideas include going on a walk to a coffee shop, making cookies together, reading a favorite magazine, listening to a new song, and visiting a friend.

Some family members create a fancy invitation, while others simply write on an index card or piece of notepaper. If you enjoy dramatic flourish and ritual, you can deliver the invites on a silver tray.

> "An invitation creates an occasion and
> adds a bright focus to the day."

Conversation Cards

Lately Colin had seemed apathetic and indifferent. Angela was tired and discouraged and having a hard time staying cheerful. Then she remembered the list she'd made at a recent care partners creativity workshop, a list of her own favorite memories, sayings, and simple pleasures.

"When the care partner is worn out, their partner senses that," Karrie Marshall says. "Creating cards with quotes, ideas, and fond memories can lift your spirits."

You can use these cards when you need a personal boost or a topic of conversation. Some care partners paste an inspiring quote, a shared memory, a line from a favorite song, or a family joke on each card. They then can share the card with the person living with dementia, using it as a conversation trigger.

After breakfast, Angela might hand Colin a card that reads, "Our weekend at the lake."

Angela tells him, "I've been thinking about the time we went to the lake, and you decided to swim across to the other side."

Colin nods in a noncommittal way; she knows he doesn't remember.

"It was before we were married," she says. "We took a picnic, and you swam across the lake and back while I watched you."

"I was a good swimmer?"

"You were and you are. You swam all during high school and kept it up all your life. In fact, we're going to the pool tomorrow."

Angela smiles as she talks to Colin about his aquatic prowess. Even though he's not saying much, he's listening. And she's enjoying talking about their shared adventures.

Creative Sparks

★ Create an invitation, asking your partner to join you for a new experience.

★ Write some favorite memories, quotes, or simple pleasures on index cards and use these cards to boost conversation with your partner.

★ Enjoy talking about your memories with your partner listening. Avoid asking, "Do you remember?" and simply share your own reminiscences.

Discover the Creativity at the End of the Rainbow

"The greater your storm, the brighter your rainbow." —Anonymous

Would you try to force a person with a broken leg to walk up three flights of stairs? No, you would find an elevator.

"We need to do the same for people living with dementia, make accommodations for their physical, mental, and psychosocial changes," says Lori La Bey, founder of Alzheimer's Speaks, which hosts a resource website, a blog, and an international radio show. "People living with memory loss are the true experts and can show us meaningful ways to support them. They have wonderful advice that goes beyond research and right to the heart of the matter."

Lori's mom lived with dementia for thirty years. Initially Lori struggled with fear of failure. As her mom's care partner, Lori was paralyzed by the terror of not doing things right. Her anxiety was fueled by limited resources and by the lack of public conversation about the disease. Looking for answers, Lori began to explore options around the world.

"People living with memory loss are the true experts and can show us meaningful ways to support them."

Understand the Pattern

Over time, Lori's mother's humor and resilience began to inspire her. Lori's dad was an enthusiastic golfer, and her mom hesitantly agreed to go with Lori to try the sport. During the outing, her mom was standing near a sand trap, club in hand. Suddenly, she fell in and when Lori rushed over to help her, she found her mom swimming the breaststroke in the sand.

"She was lying face down, moving her arms, so proud, calm, and comfortable," Lori says. "Her mind had saved her and put her in a safe place." Her mom's early lifeguard training had been triggered by the fall, and she was swimming to safety.

Then her mom broke out laughing, realizing she wasn't in her girlhood lake but in a sea of sand. Lori helped her up and all was well.

Once Lori moved beyond her fear and let in playfulness, she had many periods of deep connection with her mother.

"That was a turning point for me," Lori says. "I began to understand that she did certain things because her brain was following a pattern. I started learning not to judge and to look for the connections."

Once Lori moved beyond her fear and let in playfulness, she had many periods of deep connection with her mother. These moments were so powerful that Lori became a tireless advocate for those living with dementia and their care partners.

Talk about Dreams and Preferences

As a care partner, Lori knows it's easy to get consumed with the medical condition when someone is diagnosed with memory impairment.

"We miss out when we forget to talk to our partners about their spiritual, physical, and psychological needs," she says.

Here are some discussions Lori found to be meaningful with her own mother:

- What's on your bucket list?
- What are some of your favorite songs, singers, bands, foods, hobbies, and activities?
- Let's go through old pictures, and you can show me your favorites.
- Will you help me gather your personal history, including stories about growing up with your family, jobs you held, friends you had, sports you played, vacations you went on? This will become extremely helpful later as the disease progresses, and it will be fun to do together now.
- Shall we talk about some of our favorite moments together?
- What is important to you in your daily routine? Reading the newspaper, sipping a morning cup of coffee, taking an afternoon walk, doing a crossword puzzle?
- Would you be willing to share your experience as it progresses via writing, video, or photos, or just talking to me about it? Your insights would really help me and the rest of the family understand what you are going through.

"Dementia is a vibrant disease, encompassing the colors of the rainbow," Lori says. "If we regard it in strict black and white, we only see right or wrong. We need to let in the color and light."

Creative Sparks

★ Let go of any fears that you "won't get it right." The only misstep is if you don't try to help a person living with dementia. This is a game of trial and error, not wins and losses.

★ Talk about dreams, goals, memories, and preferences together.

★ Support your partner by adapting to the changes he is experiencing. Ask for his advice when possible.

CHAPTER FOUR

Tune In with Music and Memory

Music Matters

Fly to the Moon with Music Therapy

Embrace the Duet of Music and the Brain

Come Alive with Personal Playlists

Sing Along and Find Your Voice

Weave In Rhythm

Unearth Life's Lyrics

Encore

Music Matters

"Music expresses that which cannot be put into words
and that which cannot remain silent." —Victor Hugo

During my mom's dementia journey, music often inspired and connected us. Here is one of those melodic moments, in a paraphrased excerpt from my book, *Love in the Land of Dementia: Finding Hope in the Caregiver's Journey.* The story is set in my mom's memory care community.

Rochelle, the activity director, sticks in another tape and soon "Stardust" is playing.

"Let's dance," she says, motioning everyone to stand.

Mom looks up, and I offer her my hand.

"Want to dance?" I ask her.

"What?"

"Want to dance?" I repeat, making a swirling motion.

"What else," she says, standing up.

My parents have danced to this song many times, my mother coaxing my father onto the dance floor. I hold hands with Mom and move back and forth to the music. She laughs and does the same. I twirl her, and she walks around in a jaunty little circle. For a moment, her energy and charm have returned. I feel like I have found my long-lost mother. If my father were here, he would not be surprised. He is certain she will return to him and takes every word, every gesture of affection, every smile as a sign of hope.

"Hope is everything," Dad told me just last week. "I find something hopeful and I milk it for all it's worth. If it doesn't work out, then I search for something else. Otherwise, I am in despair."

I twirl my mom again. It is actually our first real dance together . . . .

From dancing to creating personal playlists, this chapter sings with music and rhythm-related ideas. According to numerous studies, music improves the lives of those living with dementia by reducing the need for psychotropic drugs, increasing socialization, and relieving depression.

Fly to the Moon with Music Therapy

"Where words fail, music speaks." —Hans Christian Andersen

Mollie is not in the mood to sing. Her mouth is in scowl position as she slumps onto our sofa and says, "I wish I could die."

Mollie has been wishing this for some months, but despite her ninety-seven years of life and difficulty in seeing and hearing, despite the maddening encroachment of forgetfulness and confusion, despite increased frailty and physical decline, Mollie lives on.

I sit beside Mollie, holding her one-year-old great-granddaughter Annabelle. At the sight of Annabelle's rosy cheeks and winning smile, Mollie says, "What a pretty baby. How old is she now?"

"One year," I tell her.

My life partner Ron, Mollie's son, brings Mollie a tissue and a glass of water. A knock on the door and Emily, the music therapist, comes in. She sets down her guitar case and reintroduces herself to Mollie. "We met a couple of weeks ago," she says. "I sang you songs, and we talked about your travels."

"Whatever," Mollie says, shrugging.

"Shall I sing more songs today?" Emily asks.

"If you want to," Mollie says, closing her eyes.

For the last two months, we've added a hospice team to the assisted living staff who care for Mollie. Emily is part of their arts program, and Ron and I want to experience this session with Mollie, thinking it will be something meaningful to share.

Emily has brought an array of bells and rattles. As Emily plays "Down by the Old Mill Stream," Annabelle eagerly takes two strings of bells and shakes them. Mollie's eyes are still closed, but Annabelle looks right at Emily.

"Mollie, would you like to hear 'Just the Way You Look Tonight' or 'Fly Me to the Moon'?" Emily asks.

Mollie doesn't respond, and I figure she's fallen asleep. I am about to request, "Just the Way You Look Tonight," when Mollie pipes up, her eyes still shut.

"Fly Me to the Moon,'" she says.

Emily's voice is sweet and melodic; Ron and I can't resist singing along, humming around the lyrics we've forgotten and skirting the high notes. Annabelle moves on to mini-rain sticks, adding in a soothing percussion.

You've flown a lot of places, haven't you Mollie?" Emily asks, when the song is over.

"I have." Mollie opens her eyes. "I've been around."

"You've been to France and England, is that right?"

"And India and Russia," Mollie says.

"Mom's also traveled to China, years ago, when few Americans were going there," Ron tells us.

"You've led an adventurous life," Emily says.

"I really have."

"What shall I play next? Would you like to hear 'I Left My Heart in San Francisco' or 'Oh What a Beautiful Mornin''?"

"'San Francisco.'" Mollie sits up; she and Annabelle both look at Emily as she sings the nostalgic tune.

"That's a city I'd like to visit some day," Emily says, resting her guitar across her lap. "Have you been there?"

"Many times," Mollie says.

Song by song, story by story, the hour unfolds. Emily quietly offers a choice of old standards, and the soothing familiar tunes lead into a pleasant reminiscence.

At the end of the session, Annabelle is mellowed into sprawling slumber and Mollie is sitting straight and alert. For Annabelle, the music was a lullaby and for Mollie, it was an affirming wake-up call.

Embrace the Duet of Music and the Brain

"Music is what feelings sound like." —Author Unknown

Concetta Tomaino hugged her guitar close as she walked the grim corridors of the nursing home's advanced-stage dementia unit. It was 1978 and Concetta, a graduate student in music therapy at New York University, tried not to stare at the residents, many of whom were slumped on tattered sofas or tied into wheelchairs. Some were screaming; others were calling out for help.

Concetta walked into the dayroom, where many residents were gathered in a circle. She had no idea how she could connect with these people but she sat down, calmed herself, and began playing "Let Me Call You Sweetheart" on her guitar. As she sang, something fascinating happened: The people who were agitated calmed down. Those who seemed catatonic woke up and began singing along. Concetta wondered, *How can people with such severe cognitive brain damage respond so quickly to music?*

The Power of Music

Early on, Concetta met Oliver Sacks, the neurologist and author who'd observed an amazing awakening triggered by music with his Parkinson's patients. She asked herself, *How about people living with dementia? Why do they respond to music? Can we use music to maintain or even retrieve brain function?*

These questions fueled her research and inspired her pioneering work in music therapy and the use of familiar songs with people living with end-stage dementia. She earned a doctorate in music therapy and was a founder of the Institute for Music and Neurologic Function (IMNF). This internationally recognized nonprofit offers music therapy programs to restore, maintain, and improve people's physical, emotional, and neurological function.

> "We believe music has unique powers to heal, rehabilitate, and inspire."

Concetta and other researchers discovered a strong link between music, emotions, and memory. The human brain's auditory cortex is connected to the limbic system, which processes emotions and controls various aspects of memory. Areas of the brain associated with long-term memory and emotions connect quickly with sound.

"We believe music has unique powers to heal, rehabilitate, and inspire," Concetta says. "We're trying to understand how the melodies reach areas of the brain so we can create programs that draw out the fullest function, even when there is complex neurologic damage."

Why Music Matters

According to Concetta, music is an art form people associate with major life moments. We link songs to historical and personal events. The associated memories and feelings are preserved and evoked when we hear those tunes again.

"We may forget facts, but we never lose feelings and associations," she explains. "Shared music can forge a sense of connection between people. Care partners can experiment to see which songs mean the most to their partners and why."

Even when people are nonverbal, the right tunes can lead to deep moments of bonding and can create a sense of belonging.

Using a Big Band to Move Forward

Here is how one care partner used favorite songs to connect with and soothe his beloved wife:

David was dedicated to caring for Arla at home. But getting her to take a bath was becoming increasingly difficult. He simply could not coax her out of her chair and into the bathroom. He thought back on their life together, trying to figure out what could motivate her to move. Then he remembered listening to Duke Ellington's big band. Arla loved the Duke, and she was always the first one out on the dance floor. David put on one of Ellington's CDs, and as the orchestra swelled, he held out his arms. Arla smiled and stood right up, seeming to float into his embrace. He had to grin as he danced her into the bathroom to the sound of the Duke playing, "Don't Get Around Much Anymore." Two days later, "It Don't Mean a Thing (If It Ain't Got That Swing)" came to his rescue. Day after day, the Duke inspired David's "Satin Doll" to dance her way to the bathroom.

> "Besides reducing agitation, research shows that music improves memory. I have yet to meet someone who isn't responsive to the right music."

"Besides reducing agitation, research shows that music improves memory," Concetta says. "I have yet to meet someone who isn't responsive to the right music."

Creative Sparks

★ Put together a catalogue of songs your partner likes and a list of family and friends the music connects her to. If the grandchildren are visiting, and Grandma used to take the kids to Disney movies, play or sing those Disney tunes. With adult children, revisit favorite childhood melodies.

★ Take advantage of conversational openings the lyrics might inspire. For example, if your partner asks, "When is Dad coming?" after hearing a song from his teenage years, ask, "Are you thinking about your dad? Did he like this song? Did you ever sing to it together?"

★ Seek community concerts and dementia-friendly singing groups.

★ Invite friends to share relevant songs.

★ Explore opportunities to engage with music therapists.

★ To reduce resistance and increase a feeling of safety, sing during daily care routines, such as bathing or getting ready for bed.

★ Use music, along with dancing and singing, to reduce anxiety.

★ Create your own personal playlist and share it with friends and family; listening to these songs is a wonderful way to relax and stay connected with yourself and your own history.

Come Alive with Personal Playlists

"To love a person is to learn the song that is in their heart, / And to sing it to them when they have forgotten." —Arne Garborg

Just an hour earlier, Henry was staring vacantly at the television set in the memory care unit. Now Henry is grooving, feet tapping, fingers snapping, head bobbing. His headphones block out distractions, and he hums along, blissfully engaged in his favorite songs from the 1940s.

Henry is one of thousands of people who benefit from MUSIC & MEMORY^SM, which is now used throughout the world.

Seeking Musical Solutions

One afternoon in 2006, Dan Cohen, a social worker with a background in high-tech training and software applications, was listening to a radio show that discussed the MP3 player phenomenon. As he listened, Dan wondered, *Would I have access to my favorite sixties music if I ever needed to live in a nursing home?*

He searched online and found no care facilities using MP3 players for their residents. He visited a home in Long Island, met with several residents, and learned about their favorite songs. Then he returned home, used an online music store to compile a personal playlist for each person, and loaded a few MP3 players with these preferred tunes. Back at the care home, he offered each resident head phones, and turned on their MP3 players. The results were instantaneous: they smiled and swayed as they listened to their treasured melodies.

Dan then wondered, *Would this idea work with someone who has dementia?*

Becoming Alive Inside

The answer was a resounding yes.

Dan began visiting memory care communities and working with residents, families, and staff to develop personal playlists. With a grant from the Shelley and Donald Rubin Foundation, he launched a pilot program in four care homes.

The staff reported that the Music & Memory program helped reduce anxiety, agitation, depression, and resistance to care. This meant residents needed fewer antianxiety, antipsychotic, and antidepressant medications.

Dietary staff used the music if residents stopped feeding themselves, and some began eating again. The playlists helped residents soldier through physical rehabilitation therapy. Not only did the playlists trigger memories, the songs also made people more social. Family members used the songs as icebreakers for grandchildren and as a catalyst for conversation and impromptu sing-alongs. The melodies served as a link between the generations and gave everyone a common focus.

The staff reported that the Music & Memory program helped reduce anxiety, agitation, depression, and resistance to care. This meant residents needed fewer antianxiety, antipsychotic, and antidepressant medications.

Timeless Tunes That Transcend

Barrick Wilson of Wichita, Kansas, used music to connect with his beloved wife Kristi during her dementia journey. He often took Kristi for a ride, and they'd listen to favorite songs as they tooled along.

"'Bad, Bad Leroy Brown' was one of her highlights," Barrick says.

In the afternoons, they'd sit on the sofa and sing along to golden oldies. When Barrick learned about the Roth Project: Music Memories, which is based on Music & Memory, he signed up Kristi.

"Our staff counsels care communities and families on when and how to use the music," says Linsey Norton, who served as the Alzheimer's Association's Program Director. "We also help care partners notice behavioral cues so they can reach for the headphones instead of the antianxiety medication."

Working with the Central and Western Kansas office of the Alzheimer's Association, Barrick set out to develop a playlist that keyed in on Kristi's emotional memories.

"I purchased a boxed set of Rogers and Hammerstein's Broadway musicals, records her parents had listened to at home when Kristi was growing up," Barrick says.

He used selections from the Association's extensive CD library, noting songs Kristi might have listened to from ages fifteen to twenty-five, as well as other tunes that could trigger a positive emotional connection. He added in Kristi's grandmother's favorite hymns. Volunteers loaded his selections onto an MP3 player. Then Barrick had the pleasure of sitting next to his beloved and reveling in her beautiful smile when she put on headphones and heard "Some Enchanted Evening."

Music helped Kristi when she needed to transition to a care home. The staff offered her favorite songs several times a day, and Kristi always got up and danced when "Leroy Brown" came on.

During their courtship, Barrick had serenaded Kristi on the piano in her parents' living room. When she moved into the care setting, Barrick sat at the home's piano, his wife by his side, and played "I'm in the Mood for Love," "If I Loved You," and "My Funny Valentine." These classic ballads transcended rational thought and created an engineering marvel, a bridge that connected Barrick and Kristi.

The Therapeutic Power of Favorite Tunes

For those living with dementia, Music & Memory programs include a free headset and an MP3 player programmed with favorite tunes.

"The program is therapeutic," Linsey explains. "We look at how music can contribute to the person's happiness and ease any difficult behaviors."

Results can be stunning. People tap their toes, move to the rhythm, and sing along. A man who rifles through drawers calms down while listening to favorite John Philip Sousa marches. A woman who constantly moans in pain forgets her discomfort when she hears "My Blue Heaven," a cherished love song. Even people in the end stages of dementia can connect to their meaningful melodic moments.

The Beat Goes On

"There's no downside to the music.
The program is transforming lives."

Dan Cohen invited filmmaker Michael Rossato-Bennett to capture what he was seeing on film. The result is the heart-opening documentary *Alive Inside: A Story of Music and Memory,* which won the Sundance Audience Award in 2014. Through this film, the viewer experiences the transformative powers of music for those living with dementia. Dan's goal is to have the Music & Memory program available in every nursing home, memory care community, assisted living facility, adult day center, and other places where elders live. He's also working with hospices, hospitals, and home health organizations.

"There's no downside to the music," Dan says. "The program is transforming lives."

Creative Sparks

★ To create a playlist, do a little detective work to find out what kinds of uplifting music will stimulate your partner to sing along and dance around. Learn what they listened to, when, and what the tunes meant. Ask other friends and family members to contribute ideas.

★ To test out titles, visit online music stores and play the free snippets to see what kind of reactions you get.

★ Buy an MP3 player and start downloading important songs. Share the evolving playlist with family and friends. Buy headsets to minimize distractions.

★ For support in loading the MP3 player and using the program, contact the Alzheimer's Association or the Music & Memory program.

★ Purchase a splitter, which plugs into two MP3 players, so you can listen together.

★ Ask yourself: How can this tool improve our lives?
Are there times of day when the playlist might make
life easier for your partner? Are there times you can
listen together? Are there times you need a few quiet
moments? The personal playlist can serve any or all of
these purposes.

★ When your partner is ready to listen, help him put
on the headphones. Turn on the songs and watch for
reactions. Try the playlist several times, noting the
refrains that sizzle and those that fizzle. Then adjust
accordingly.

★ Be ready to discuss memories that flood out.

★ If the program doesn't work perfectly the first time,
don't give up. You may just need to change the songs.

Sing Along and Find Your Voice

"I don't sing because I'm happy;
I'm happy because I sing." —William James

During the first sing-along, Frank drifted near the table of
singers, pausing while they crooned "Que Sera, Sera." He then
moved on, striding the corridors, peering out the windows, pacing
back down the hallway, and into the community room again. At
the next week's sing-along at Pacifica Memory Care Unit in
Santa Fe, New Mexico, Jytte Lokvig, PhD, handed out the bright

orange folders thick with popular songs of an earlier era and again invited Frank to join them. He kept wandering. But he did drop by for "Goodnight Irene."

The following week, as always, Jytte offered Frank a songbook, which he actually opened and looked at.

"Won't you join us?" she asked.

> "Singing together creates community.
> Even those who don't sing are positively
> impacted by the energy of the music."

Frank sat down and joined in when they belted out "She'll Be Coming 'Round the Mountain" and "You Are My Sunshine." Within two months, Frank was at the table before Jytte arrived, waiting eagerly to add his voice to the chorus.

"Singing together creates community," Jytte explains to me, when I visit her sing-along. "Even those who don't sing are positively impacted by the energy of the music."

Soaring through Singing

Jytte is the author of *The Alzheimer's Creativity Project* and an expert in creating enrichment and activities for people living with dementia. I met her through a telephone interview and wanted to experience her magic in person. So, on a visit to Santa Fe, I sat in on a singing session. I instantly felt the sense of community as I settled between Jytte and Edwin at a long table in the home's common area. Edwin, a resident, shared his book with me. He knew all the lyrics and really seemed to enjoy being part of the group. Several chairs away, Bette was sighing and shaking her hands, then calling out in a high-pitched voice. She made a squeaky noise, then giggled.

During a break in the music, Edwin told me, "Bette and I speak the same language. You won't believe what goes on between us."

Larry also knew all the words. When Jytte lingered between songs, Larry kept things rolling by starting the next number.

Celia was in her early fifties and didn't like to sit still. Though she didn't speak, her desire for closeness was apparent in her beautiful smile and her willingness to hover around the singers. As we sang "True Love," Celia walked by and looked into my eyes. I gazed into hers, and she mouthed a few words, then moved on.

Twenty tunes later, the energy in the room was rich with laughter, companionship, and excitement.

Music Opens the Doorway to Creative Expression

Jytte believes that music is a doorway to creating connections.

"Even when I do an art activity, I start with a few songs to knit us together," she says.

Bringing singing into your daily life is a simple way to connect with yourself and with the person you're caring for. You can start by discussing the kinds of music you both enjoy.

"Don't forget to include silly or humorous ditties," Jytte says. "Too much lost love and heartbreak can be depressing."

Once you have a working list, print lyrics in large type and create a songbook for each participant.

"The songbook is a symbol of the group, even if it's a group of two," Jytte says. "It means you belong."

Bringing singing into your daily life is a simple way to connect with yourself and with the person you're caring for.

Creative Sparks

★ Give yourself permission to belt it out even if you can't hit every note.

★ Sing with gusto and enjoy large gestures and eye contact.

★ Use the music to stimulate conversation.

★ Enjoy creating ritual by singing the same selections over and over. If you find certain choices aren't sparking energy, omit them and discuss adding others.

★ Clap at the end of each song, giving yourselves a round of applause.

★ Invite others to join you. Include family members, friends, and anyone else who's willing to sing.

★ Sometimes the singing flows and other times, it doesn't. Tune in and be ready to change the song list.

Weave In Rhythm

"Anytime you strike the drums, you have to be aware that you're creating a musical event." —Vinnie Colaiuta

At age twenty-two, Marlon Sobol was ready to change the world through drumming. His parents were both musicians and his mother had used music with children who had special, needs. It was natural that Marlon should gravitate toward music therapy. That spring 2002, Marlon started as a music specialist in a dementia unit in White Plains, New York. He had no training in dementia but figured he could learn.

Marlon planned to go in with his drum and magically engage all the residents. He got off the elevator onto the fifth floor unit, a small goblet-shaped West African drum over his shoulder, and immediately began smiling and drumming.

"A resident wheeled up to me and dug her nails into the back side of my hand while I was drumming," Marlon recalls. "She was basically telling me to leave."

Marlon had never considered that the rhythmic pounding might agitate and confuse people.

"I realized I needed to get to know the residents before I offered them something new," he says.

Now, as a staff music therapist at the Institute for Music and Neurologic Function (IMNF) in White Plains, New York, Marlon helps people with dementia and other cognitive issues connect with themselves through rhythmic activities using percussion instruments, chanting, and movement.

Use Rhythm as a Meeting Point

Even when people have memory issues, their lives still have rhythm. Their heartbeat, breathing, and walking are rhythmic. Their daily schedules typically have a regular cadence.

"Rhythmic movements boost communication, reduce anxiety, improve mood, and enhance motor skills," Marlon says. "They offer a safe way to express emotions and create music."

Drumming lets people produce meaningful sounds even when their communication skills have deteriorated. The shared tempo offers a connection that goes beyond rational functioning and verbal abilities. Some people get out of their chairs and dance. Others stomp their feet and snap their fingers, while others simply move their heads and sway.

"Regardless of their level of movement, they are engaged in a full expression of life," Marlon says.

> "Rhythmic movements boost communication, reduce anxiety, improve mood, and enhance motor skills."

Communicate through Drumming

Marlon often begins a session with familiar music that has a strong beat. The components often include chanting, singing, and shaking, or hitting percussion instruments. Marlon adds motion—shaking to the right, to the left, up and down, and to the center—and encourages people to experiment.

"What if we hit the drum with our palms?" he might ask. "How does it sound if we tap with our fingers?"

He may model shaking the maracas in circles and then moving them side-to-side like windshield wipers. He invites rapid movements, then slower motions. He encourages people to play loudly, then to make mellow sounds. Throughout the experience, he reinforces people's actions, stating, "Wow! Did you hear the sound you just made?"

Creative Sparks

★ You don't need to be musical to enjoy and benefit from rhythmic activities.

★ Offer a choice of percussion instruments. You can use homemade noisemakers, such as banging a pot with spoons, hitting a pen on a book, or shaking a container filled with beans. You can also simply tap your hands on your knees or a tabletop.

★ Play familiar tunes with a steady beat and moderate tempo.

★ Invite movement, then encourage and appreciate the sounds, including your own. Comment on how the sounds contribute to the experience.

★ Explore communicating through call and response drumming. One of you taps out a beat, and the other answers. It's another way to have a conversation.

★ Model the movements. Even when people are unable
to play instruments, they can still participate through
movements, gestures, facial expressions, sounds, and
eye contact.

Unearth Life's Lyrics

"Music and rhythm find their way into the
secret places of the soul." —Plato

The song "What Do You Do with a Drunken Sailor?" might
seem out of place in a memory care community. But an elder
requested it so musician Judith-Kate Friedman strums her guitar
and sings the folk song. Many of the elders chime in for the
chorus. It's the beginning of a two-hour Songwriting Works™
session, and Judith-Kate has already connected with each person.
Some family members and staff are also attending the workshop.

After the rousing first song, Judith-Kate asks people about
their favorite types of music. She invites the group to take some
deep breaths together. Then she guides them in a warm-up, which
includes clapping out rhythms, making noises, such as *ahhhs* and
oooohs and singing a favorite tune, such as "This Little Light of
Mine," "This Land Is Your Land," or "Home on the Range." She
smiles and laughs, inviting people to go beyond any shyness and
join in the fun.

Judith-Kate is a professional musician with a background
in ethnomusicology and folklore. Since 1990, she has been

facilitating Songwriting Works™ for a variety of populations. One of her songwriting programs serves people who are living with dementia and other cognitive issues, along with their care partners.

Theresa Allison, MD, M. Music, made a nine-month study of the Songwriting Works™ method, tracking forty elders who composed both secular and sacred music. Dr. Allison found that "creating and performing original songs enabled institutionalized elders to remain vibrant and creative despite the progression of physical and cognitive challenges."

Judith-Kate now asks the group, "Who has written a song before?"

No one answers.

"Who has an idea for a song? What should we write about?" Judith-Kate asks. Then she assures the group, "All ideas are good; there's no wrong answer."

Dr. Allison found that "creating and performing original songs enabled institutionalized elders to remain vibrant and creative despite the progression of physical and cognitive challenges."

A staff member stands beside a large pad, ready to write. Everyone—elders, family, staff, and volunteers—is encouraged to throw in suggestions.

"I want to write about sending my grandkid to the moon," one woman offers.

"My favorite meal," says another.

"Christmas."

The ideas flow, and Judith-Kate notes each topic on the easel.

"I'd like to write a love song."

"I'd like to write about going to the beach in the summer."

"I used to go to the beach every summer."

"I was at the beach when a hurricane was near."

As the brainstorming session progresses, Judith-Kate makes sure each person is included, again and again. Every suggestion seems to trigger another.

"Repetition works in everyone's favor," Judith-Kate says.

Design the Lyrics through Stoking Stories

Though Judith-Kate has worked primarily with groups, family care partners can easily use her ideas at home.

During each of Judith-Kate's songwriting sessions, stories emerge. In another memory care community, a woman talks about riding an elephant, describing the view. Veterans discuss their World War II memories. One man says, "I was with my twin brother in the Marines. We went all over the world, and we both came home, alive." He talks about traveling to the Philippines on the big ship, their wives waiting for them, and the joyous homecoming celebrations. Several other veterans speak of their wartime experiences, and the group weaves the individual stories into the song. Over the course of the workshop, their sentences get longer, and they engage more.

Judith-Kate has learned that participants often blossom when they have enough time to express themselves. "People who are living with dementia are often more capable than many realize. In order to appreciate their abilities—and gifts—we need to allow enough time for connection and participation," Judith-Kate says. "The benefits of this creative process include new friendships and stronger communication and cooperation."

The scribe records every word, and Judith-Kate reads all the ideas to the group. Then comes the moment to find a melody and a theme that can bind these colorful ideas into a song.

"People who are living with dementia are
often more capable than many realize."

"We're trying to create a melody that is memorable and singable," Judith-Kate says. The results range from songs about war and peace to anthems about home to stories about family. The songs are often hauntingly real and beautiful, rich with personal imagery, emotion, and drama.

Why Songwriting Works

You don't need to be a singer or musician to get started with songwriting. You just need to be willing to experiment.

"We encourage and include wild ideas," Judith-Kate says. "Composing a song from scratch can be initially intimidating, but it's ultimately liberating."

You don't need to be a singer or musician
to get started with songwriting. You just
need to be willing to experiment.

Creative Sparks

Each of these ideas can be its own session, or you can combine ideas for a songwriting flow.

★ Take a breath, then press your lips together and make an "mmmm" sound.

★ Clap out a rhythm to something you've said. For example, you can clap out, "The dog lies in the sun." This makes the idea of rhythm tangible, and it's also silly and fun. You can clap along to any phrase or sentence.

★ Explore topics by asking, "What shall we write a song about?" Use pictures to jump-start the process. If your songwriting partner adores her dog, you might show a photo of the pet and ask for some favorite stories about the pet.

★ If needed, come up with your own suggestions.

★ Write down every word either of you say. Ask questions to expand the conversation.

★ Read aloud all the ideas and experiment with putting your words to a melody.

★ Feel free to use a familiar tune to get started; the fun is in the flow of music and words. Then dare to improvise, sing, whistle, or tap out a brand-new tune!

★ Share your creation with others. Make a recording or video and email it to friends and family or invite a few musical friends to round out the sound and add depth to the singing experience.

Encore

"A song will outlive all sermons
in the memory." —Henry Giles

Tune In without the Word

"Humming offers a soothing vibration in your mouth," says Teepa Snow, a leading dementia care educator and developer of Positive Approach™ to Care. "When you hum, you take someone who's all alone and bring them along with you."

When you hum, you invite interaction. People don't need to worry about forgetting the words. Plus you breathe more deeply when you hum.

Name that Tune

"If people lose speech, make up a song, repeating their name, so they know it's them," says Magdalena Schamberger, Chief Executive and Artistic Director, Hearts & Minds. "When you're singing, stroke their arm in time to the song."

Soundscapes

"Think of pleasant sounds, such as children laughing, steaks sizzling, ocean waves, or birds singing," says Mara Botonis, author of *When Caring Takes Courage: A Compassionate, Interactive Guide for Alzheimer's and Dementia Caregivers.* "These sounds can spark up an activity. You can download these from the Internet or find a themed CD."

CHAPTER FIVE

Add Imagination to Movement

Explore Creative Movement and Exercise

Ah-Ha-Ha with Laughter

Brighten the Brain with Movement Therapy

Work Wonders with Workouts

Partner Dancing for a Purpose

Explore Creative Movement and Exercise

"I move, therefore I am." —Haruki Murakami

During my mother's journey, my dad was determined to keep her moving—walking, swimming, and gardening. He was determined to move her through her confusion.

My father intuitively understood the importance of exercise. Significant global research shows that exercise can slow both the onset and the advancement of dementia. That means walking, stretching, deep breathing, laughing, and dancing are good for both the care partner and the person living with dementia.

Jeff Burns, MD, Codirector of the University of Kansas's Alzheimer's Disease Center, is one of the researchers studying the impact of exercise on the brain, with a goal of learning how to prevent, delay, or slow the advancement of dementia.

"We view exercise as medicine," he says. "Our observational studies show that people who exercise perform better on cognitive tests, have healthier brains on their brain scans, and show a lower long-term risk of developing dementia."

Dr. Burns's research looked at different doses of exercise and noted cognitive benefits for those exercising only seventy-five minutes per week. The group that worked out for 225 minutes every week enjoyed even greater cognitive levels.

"A little movement brings benefits, but more is better," he says.

In this section, experts offer imaginative and fun "step by step by step" ideas for moving into a happier and healthier space.

"We view exercise as medicine. Our observational studies show that people who exercise perform better on cognitive tests, have healthier brains on their brain scans, and show a lower long-term risk of developing dementia."

Ah-Ha-Ha with Laughter

"When you laugh, you change, and when you change, the whole world changes."
—Madan Kataria, MD, Founder of Laughter Yoga Movement

There's no speaker standing on stage making witty remarks. There is no video showing humorous stories and no comical music playing in the background. Yet the meeting room is packed with business people pretending they're having hilarious cell phone conversations and laughing uproariously. In the middle of the room, chuckling wildly, is Madan Kataria, MD, the founder of the internationally acclaimed Laughter Yoga movement. This session is one of thousands of Laughter Club meetings worldwide, where people come together for the purpose of happiness and healing through a series of playful, accessible, and profound laughter exercises.

Laughing Matters

"Laughing is a skill anyone can master, and laughter yoga is ideal for people living with dementia," says Madan. "Laughter yoga is an aerobic workout that helps uplift your mood within minutes by releasing endorphins from your brain cells. You often remain energized, relaxed, and in good spirits throughout the day. You will probably laugh more than you normally do."

> Laughter improves blood circulation and increases the net amount of oxygen to body and brain, which makes us feel more healthy and energetic. Laughter also makes our immune system stronger.

Madan explains that the brain requires 25 percent more oxygen than other organs. Laughter is like an exhalation; it removes residual air from lungs and increases oxygenation. A rise in brain oxygen helps sharpen memory and helps relieve depression and anxiety. Laughter improves blood circulation and increases the net amount of oxygen to body and brain, which makes us feel more healthy and energetic. Laughter also makes our immune system stronger. If you laugh regularly you will not fall sick easily, and if you have chronic health conditions they will heal faster. Plus laughing with others builds a social bond and reduces feelings of isolation.

Madan created a unique routine that combines laughter exercises with yoga breathing and allows anyone to laugh.

"This is about exercise, not real laughter," Madan says.

No Jokes Necessary when Learning to Laugh

When Madan first gathered together a few people in Mumbai, India, to start a laughter club, they relied on jokes and funny stories for sources of merriment. But they soon ran out of humorous tales. Madan researched the science of laughter and learned that when you laugh voluntarily, the body does not differentiate between fake and real hilarity. You receive the same physiological and psychological advantages. He also discovered that you need at least ten to fifteen minutes of continuous laughter to truly receive the health benefits. He began developing the four tenets of his groundbreaking program: physical movements and gestures, breathing practice, child-like playfulness, and laughter exercises.

Since he founded the program in 1995, he has practiced daily, sustained laughter. Because of laughter yoga, Madan believes his immune system is stronger; and in all those years, he has not experienced a cold, cough, or sore throat. He has become increasingly mentally positive and easily flows through challenges. He also feels he has an increased capacity to help others.

Ha Ha Warm-Ups

Ideally, Madan suggests a small group for your laughter exercises. But laughing also works solo and one-on-one. Start by telling your partner about the concrete benefits of laughing and the fun of making yourselves laugh.

Then demonstrate an initial warm up, saying clearly, "Ho ho ho" and "Ha ha ha." With each syllable, clap your hands and invite your partner to talk and clap along. Add movements, clapping to the left, then the right, holding your hands up, then down. You can add to the syllables, including "hee hee hees" and "tee hee hees."

Singing is also a great way to warm up. Madan recommends the Ha Ha chorus, which simply substitutes "ha ha" for the lyrics of any song. So, belt out "Happy Birthday to You" by simply singing, "Ha ha ha ha ha ha" to the tune. Don't be surprised if all the ha-ha-ing makes you giggle.

"Laughing, singing, dancing, and playing are the elements of joy," Madan says. "The world is a difficult place, and it's easy to get depressed. That's why it's important to fill your blood with positive chemistry through breathing, stretching, and laughing."

The Scintillating Science of Laughing

Carmela Carlyle chants, "Ho ho ha ha ha," clapping her hands to the rhythm of the words. The circle of elders follow suit. Carmela puts her hands on her middle and says, "Now let's have a big belly laugh." She shakes her belly with her hands as her laughter erupts. The elders, who have diverse levels of dementia, echo her with their own belly laughs. Carmela points at herself and says, "If we laugh at ourselves, we will never run out of material."

Laughter Is Too Serious to Rely on Jokes

Initially some families worry about their partners looking silly or crazy, sitting around, guffawing for no reason. Carmela, who is a dementia care specialist, certified laughter yoga teacher, and the creator of the training DVD *Laughter Yoga with Elders*, reassures them, saying, "We get physically fit by going to the gym and 'pretending' to run on the treadmill. This 'pretend' laughter develops brain cells and alters our biochemistry."

"Research from the neuroscience community shows us the brain is not static. Through laughter, we can develop brain cells and lay down new neurosynapses," Carmela says. "When we laugh, our jaws move, sending a message directly to the brain to release feel-good hormones. People living with dementia can bypass the intellect and go directly to the powerful medicine of laughter."

Carmela integrated laughter yoga into her life initially as a way to manage her own chronic pain from a spinal injury. In 2007, she trained to become a certified laughter yoga leader and created the Chair and Wheelchair Laughter Yoga Club.

Carmela has seen how the practice lights up people who have advanced dementia. "Sometimes people laugh for the first time in years," she says. "Laughing evokes social memories, happy times of being with friends. We are social beings, and people with dementia can connect through laughing and being around laughter."

"Research from the neuroscience community shows us the brain is not static. Through laughter, we can develop brain cells and lay down new neurosynapses."

Laughter Rx

Carmela helps families integrate laughter into their lives.

"Begin by telling your loved one that it is doctor's orders to laugh frequently," she advises. "Explain the benefits of laughter and how it is proven as good exercise."

Carmela offers ways to sprinkle laughter into the daily routine. Instead of singing in the shower, she suggests warbling the "ho ho ha ha ha" chorus and laughing while getting clean. To ease the stress of helping your partner dress, she invites laughing at each item of clothing. You might say, "The left leg is going into the pants. Ha ha ha. Right foot going into the shoe. Ha ha ha." When driving to medical appointments, Carmela likes to laugh during red lights.

"Even if your partner doesn't laugh right away, that's fine," Carmela says. "You help yourself when you laugh, and your partner benefits from the sound of hilarity."

Creative Sparks

★ Explain the scientific benefits of laughter to your partner and introduce the idea of laughing together.

★ Watch for ten-second opportunities to sprinkle laughter into your routine: Laugh when putting on shoes or brushing hair. Laugh when setting the table or walking downstairs. Laugh at red lights.

★ Sing a familiar song using only the "ha ha" syllables, such as "You Are My Sunshine." You'll probably both smile and giggle.

★ Hold two imaginary glasses of milk and pour from one to the other while making mirthful sounds. Be careful not to spill on the imaginary carpet, but be sure to laugh if you do.

★ Feeling a little irritated or out of sorts? Pretend you're jabbing at a punching bag and accompany each thrust of fist with a resounding, "Ho ho" and "Ha ha ha."

★ Wiggle around like you have ants in your pants and laugh.

★ Look at the clock and say "Let's see if we can laugh for five seconds straight!" Make it a game throughout the day.

★ Send loving giggles to a part of yourself that needs a little energy or love. Or beam laughter to a friend or loved one.

★ Use your imaginations to vary the exercises, adding in new playful scenarios.

★ Integrate laughter yoga into your visits and include family and friends.

★ Explore laughter yoga videos and soundtracks on the Internet. Join a Laughter Yoga Club in your area. There are also Skype clubs, where you can laugh with people from across the globe.

Brighten the Brain with Movement Therapy

"Movement is a medicine for creating change in a person's physical, emotional, and mental state." —Carol Welch

Seven people circle the brightly colored piece of cloth, holding its edges and shaking it to the beat of "(I Love You) For Sentimental Reasons."

"What does this fabric remind you of?" asks Natasha Goldstein-Levitas, a Philadelphia, Pennsylvania-based Registered Dance/Movement Therapist (R-DMT) who regularly works with people who live in memory care communities.

"We're shaking out a tablecloth," one woman says.

"We're hanging clothes outside to dry," says another.

"We're cutting up onions for potato salad," says another.

"When might we eat potato salad?" Natasha asks.

"A Fourth of July picnic," a man answers.

Everyone lowers the cloth to the floor, and they discuss who might be at the picnic. They mention a sister, a husband, a child, and discuss some of their favorite summer foods. When the conversation wanes, Natasha moves around the circle, offering each person a squirt of coconut-scented hand sanitizer and rubbing it into their palms. As Natasha gently massages the fragrant lotion into the hands of a woman who rarely talks, Natasha asks, "What does this fragrance remind you of?"

The woman looks right at her and says, "Hawaii."

Invite People into the Movement

"Movement therapy is based on the principle that the mind and body are connected," Natasha says. "Movement helps people feel empowered. I try to capitalize on the strengths of each person. We celebrate small successes, even if it's just making eye contact, taking deeper breaths, or saying a word."

When working with those living with memory loss, Natasha sits people in a circle, turns on music, and observes reactions.

"Music with a strong rhythm, such as Motown or Celtic, works well for people with severe dementia," she says. "I also choose music that is near and dear to them, such as hits from the 1940s or 1950s."

If people aren't clapping along or moving their foot or hand to the music, Natasha will gently tap their chair, shoulder, or hand in rhythm to get them started.

If anyone is moving his or her lips or singing along, Natasha adds her encouragement. "It looks like Carrie knows this song," she might say.

She tailors her exercises to each individual, concentrating on simple movements, such as opening and closing the fingers or stretching arms overhead. She describes every gesture and frequently reminds people to breathe deeply.

"Movement helps people feel empowered. . . . We celebrate small successes, even if it's just making eye contact, taking deeper breaths, or saying a word."

Add Imagination to Activities

Natasha might guide her group into moving their fingers and pretending to pluck grapes off the vine. Suddenly, a woman opens her hand, and all her pretend grapes fall to the ground.

"Let's stomp them and make wine out of them," a man says, and they all stomp away.

"Talking about food causes a lot of excitement. Using concrete situations, such as picking fruit, evokes cooking and eating memories," Natasha says.

Sometimes real food is added to the movement sequences. Natasha brings in a basket of clementines and asks each person to choose one. They hold the fruits, gently squeezing them. They notice how each fruit is unique. Natasha asks questions, such as "What other orange objects can you think of? What does the aroma remind you of?" While they talk, they massage their arms by rolling the clementines up and down.

For people in wheelchairs, Natasha sometimes unfurls a long rug, puts on celebratory music, and invites them to pretend they're going down the red carpet.

"The carpet serves as a structure," she explains. She uses the same structure to encourage people to walk, placing an interesting object on each end and urging people to walk to the object. In addition to physical movement, Natasha engages the senses, using textures, aromas, colors, sounds, and tastes.

"Any kind of movement can stimulate memory and creativity," Natasha says.

Creative Sparks

★ Orchestrate a calm environment without extraneous noises or distractions.

★ Put on rhythmic music at a low volume. If your partner is agitated, gently tapping her shoulders can be soothing.

★ Invite your partner to move in any way that feels right. If he's angry, suggest, "Let's stomp our feet, shake our arms, or wiggle our fingers."

★ Engage the senses by inviting your partner to hold and examine an object with texture, color, and scent, such as an orange, grapefruit, or lemon. Invite both exercise and conversation by holding cloth or scarves and moving them around together.

★ Provide a serene end to the session by smoothing fragrant lotions onto the hands. Select scents that might evoke memories, such as lavender, rose, or cinnamon.

Work Wonders with Workouts

"It is exercise alone that supports the spirits, and
keeps the mind in vigor." —Marcus Tullius Cicero

Michael Berg hands out paint stir sticks and puts on a John
Philip Sousa march.

"Let's use these sticks as an orchestra conductor's baton," he
says. Standing in the middle of the circle, Michael shows the
exercisers how to use their arms and shoulders, moving in time to
the music, incorporating ideas from Conductorcise, developed by
Maestro David Dworkin.

"Any movement is good movement. When
you use the body in new ways, you
also use the mind in new ways."

Michael Berg is Life Enhancement Coordinator at Highgate
Senior Living in Bellingham, Washington. He designed the
movement class to engage people of all abilities on a mental,
physical, and even spiritual level.

"Any movement is good movement," Michael Berg says.
"When you use the body in new ways, you also use the mind in
new ways."

Although Michael typically works with a group, these exercises
are also effective one-on-one.

Circle Up and Move

> "They have a treasure trove of experiences. If we take the time to meet them where they are, we all come away enriched."

Michael begins his sessions by issuing an invitation to move.

"I explain that people in wheelchairs get the same workout, just the sitting down version," Michael says.

Using rousing marching music, Michael encourages the exercisers to move their hips back and forth, keeping with the beat. He describes the movements and reminds people of the benefits, saying, "This is good for your thinking process. This will get the blood moving around your body. Standing and moving around is good for fall prevention."

After marching, Michael puts on mellow music as they do a further series of movement, coordination, and mime activities that involve strength, stretching, and awareness. They may play a quick teamwork game, such as passing a beach ball around the circle. Or they may create a story by going around the circle with each person saying one word.

The grand finale includes visualization with a posture designed to help right/left brain integration. People sit in their chairs with feet on the ground, ankles crossed. Their wrists are also crossed and resting in their laps. Their eyes are closed. Michael plays soft instrumental music and reminds them to breathe easily. Michael then invites them to think positive, offering an affirmation, such as, "I feel wonderful." He asks the group to repeat it after him.

When the class is over, the exercisers applaud and go to lunch happy and hungry. While the group is at lunch, Michael hands out warm towels with peppermint oil on them for cleansing and aromatherapy.

Michael has learned a great deal from those living with dementia. "They have a treasure trove of experiences," he says. "If we take the time to meet them where they are, we all come away enriched."

Bring the Exercises Home

To keep yourself fit, modify your own workout routine so you can do it with your partner. Here's an example of how that might work.

Months ago, when her sister Bess moved in, Emily gave up her morning workout. She wanted to help Bess, who struggled with cognitive impairment, get used to her new surroundings. But now Emily includes Bess in her movement routine. To accommodate Bess's energy level, Emily exercises midmorning instead of at the break of dawn. To keep herself fit, she does each exercise first, then performs it in a simpler way as she talks Bess through it. When Emily does her push-ups, Bess sits in a chair and pushes herself out of the chair using her hands. Emily does her leg lifts, then holds hands with Bess, inviting her to step over an imaginary rock with her right foot, then step with her left foot. During the process, she compliments Bess for her efforts.

Creative Sparks

★ Try different kinds of music with different styles and tempos. If music seems too stimulating, try a CD of soft forest sounds or go for silence. For continuity, use the same songs for a week.

★ Create a customized version of your own exercise
program. Do an exercise and have your partner watch.
Then do the modified version together. Describe what
parts of the body you are working and mention the
benefits.

★ End with a short visualization that invites positive
thinking.

★ Explore different kinds of physical experiences,
including balancing, aerobic, and strengthening
exercises.

Partner Dancing for a Purpose

"Dancing is the poetry of the foot." —John Dryden

Latin music sizzles throughout the room and Nathan Hescock
holds out his hand to his dance student Bea. She accepts the
invitation by putting her hand in his. He helps her out of her chair
and supports her as they move their shoulders to the rhythm. Her
eyes shine, and she sings an operatic tune in a quivering soprano.
For those moments, Bea is not just another ninety-two-year-old
with dementia. She's a beautiful woman in the arms of a handsome
man, swaying to her favorite music.

Bea and others like her were the inspiration for the New
York City-based nonprofit Rhythm Break Cares (RBC) founded

by ballroom instructor Nathan Hescock. Originally, he'd agreed to lead a six-week dance/movement class for those living with dementia at the request of the United Way. The experience was so gratifying that he kept going.

"People may lose words and the ability to recognize others, but they still have vitality, creativity, and the ability to dance," Nathan says.

In addition to working with care facilities and individuals, RBC hosts a monthly tea dance for people with dementia and their care partners.

> "People may lose words and the ability to recognize others, but they still have vitality, creativity, and the ability to dance."

"It's a very social time, filled with sweetness," Nathan says. "People with dementia are often very sensitive to others with dementia who are worse off. They'll go up, take someone's hand, and try to coax the person out of his shell. It's a very meaningful experience."

Dancing without the Stars

"Music, movement, and touch are the founding principles behind RBC," says Stine Moen, director of operations.

Although the RBC team has ballroom dancing experience, you don't need dancing skills to easily incorporate these movements at home.

Often, dance partners are initially slumped into a chair, head bent, eyes shut, mouths closed. But once the dancing begins, the lethargy evaporates.

"When you are holding your partner, bearing her weight, and moving with her, there's an electricity between you," Nathan says. "Through eye contact, rhythm, and touch, there's a joy and sense of connectedness that transcends the ability to finish a sentence."

Many clients who don't like to exercise light up when dancing.

"We dance with people in wheelchairs as well," Stine says. "We hold their hands and lead and most of them can move shoulders and upper bodies and wiggle their chests."

For those with extremely limited mobility, the instructors hold their hands and move in place while maintaining eye contact.

"Through eye contact, rhythm, and touch, there's a joy and sense of connectedness that transcends the ability to finish a sentence."

Shall We Dance?

Familiar tunes with a steady tempo and repetitive choruses work well. Elvis Presley and Frank Sinatra often get people moving. A few great dance numbers include "You Make Me Feel So Young"; "I've Got You Under My Skin"; "All Shook Up"; and "New York, New York." If your city or state is lucky enough to have a familiar song, add that to your list.

Here are some examples of the transformative powers of partner dancing.

Carmen, a dance student with advanced dementia, was one of Stine's special partners. As soon as Stine put on Elvis's "Now or Never," Carmen woke right up and got out of her chair, ready to dance.

Another student, Rex, lived in a memory community, walked with a cane, and had trouble balancing.

"I'm too old to do anything," Rex insisted.

When Stine and the instructors danced with other students, Rex scowled from the sidelines. But when they played "It Had to Be You," Rex was ready to dance. He and Stine waltzed around the room together, and in those moments, Rex was full of life.

Lead by Following

A good leader is a good follower, Nathan believes. The leader creates a safe space so dancers can express themselves physically. As a leader, you're not instructing; you're following your partner's energy.

> As a leader, you're not instructing; you're following your partner's energy.

"Flexibility is key," Stine says. "Don't plan the session too well."

Nathan and the RBC instructors know how much pleasure partner dancing brings.

"It's beautiful to see people come to life," Stine says.

Creative Sparks

★ Assess your partner's ability to move. Will she dance standing up or move rhythmically in a chair? Will you hold her or only hold her hands?

★ Play a favorite song with a steady beat and an easy-to-sing chorus.

★ Look into your partner's eyes and hold out your hand as an invitation to dance.

★ While assuming the leader's position, allow your partner to guide you, following his lead as he responds to the music.

★ Enjoy the experience, and afterward thank your partner for the dance.

CHAPTER SIX

Cook Up Memorable Moments

Create Meaningful Moments through Food

Feed Friendships by Cooking

Build Brain Power with Culinary Creativity

A Feast for the Senses

Nibble on a Few Extras

Create Meaningful Moments through Food

"Food is our common ground, a universal experience." —James Beard

The dread seizes me in early October. Thanksgiving is normally my favorite holiday, and I always look forward to seeing my parents from Memphis and my brother and his family from Chicago. But last year, Mom seemed so lost and confused. I understood she had dementia, yet I didn't fully understand all it entailed. But when Mom showed up without her famous date crumbs, butterscotch brownies, and bourbon balls, I knew everything had changed. Despite my mother's sweet attitude, seeing her clenched hands and tight mouth broke my heart.

This year, I vow things will be different. I will find ways to engage Mom and to deal with my own expectations and emotions. I start by asking my brother Dan if he can bake Mom's date crumbs. Being a nice guy and a great cook, he agrees.

Then I explore ways Mom can still contribute to the meal. Dan is head chef, and I am sous-chef. I decide to include Mom in the vegetable preparation, and my parents join me at the dining room table. I remind Mom how to snap green beans, and she sits beside me, contentedly breaking beans. Then we take dull dinner knives and slice mushrooms. My father supervises, eating cashews and reminiscing.

"Fran, remember our first Thanksgiving together?" he asks.

Mom smiles. I call my brother into the room; I know he loves hearing this old story.

"Manchester," she says.

"That's right. We lived in a little apartment in Manchester, New Hampshire. It was before Deborah was born."

"I ruined our oven."

Dad beams and waits to hear if Mom has more to say. She looks at him expectantly, and he continues the story.

"Fran had been in the kitchen all morning," Dad says. "Right before our guests arrived, we heard a loud popping sound. Fran rushed into the kitchen, and I was right behind her. The oven was splattered with turkey and dressing, and the bones of the bird were just about bare. Fran had left the innards in the turkey, sewed it shut, and it exploded. We had a vegetarian Thanksgiving that year."

"What a great story," Dan says. "I think of that every time I roast a turkey."

"You're a good cook," Mom says.

We resume our mushroom slicing. Mom seems at ease, which means that Dad is also relaxed. Next we fold napkins together.

Then I bring in fruit; Mom picks grapes off their stems and transfers blueberries and raspberries into a big salad bowl.

That afternoon, friends join us for our Thanksgiving feast. When they praise the meal, I introduce the sous team and am pleased to include Mom. Mom smiles, and I take her hand.

"Did I help?" she quietly asks.

"You sure did."

"I'm glad," she says. "I always like to help."

My brother carries in a tray of sweets; he's baked all our favorites. Mom picks a date crumb and a butterscotch brownie.

"These are good," she says, smiling.

"They ought to be," I say. "They're your recipes."

Kitchen Connections

"The act of preparing food can draw on long-term memory and trigger activities people have done in the past."

"Cooking together can help family members connect in the kitchen," says Kate Pierce, LMSW, Alzheimer's Association Greater Michigan Chapter. "The act of preparing food can draw on long-term memory and trigger activities people have done in the past."

As a care partner, you may need to make meals, so working together in the kitchen offers a low-stress way to accomplish a task and relive family and food memories. People want to be useful, and Kate believes creating meals for and with someone meets that need.

For a successful experience, Kate offers these tips:

- When designing cooking activities, consider your partner's current skills. Make sure the number of steps is appropriate to the level of memory loss.
- Set up a quiet environment with few distractions.
- Set out the food and utensils, so everything is at the ready. If possible, use the same type of equipment your partner used in the past.
- Offer as much independence as possible and be ready to help as needed.

Creative Sparks

★ Select a treasured recipe or favorite food.

★ Choose simple, safe tasks you can do together. Examples include snapping beans, tearing lettuce for a salad, separating orange slices, or mixing nuts and raisins. You might also enjoy washing and drying dishes together.

★ Use the foods, the preparation, or the occasion as a catalyst for conversation and reminiscing. Encourage stories and ask open-ended questions.

★ Look for seasonal recipes or foods that have delicious aromas, interesting textures, or evoke good memories. Some examples include baking holiday cookies, preparing cinnamon rolls, mashing potatoes, or cranking ice cream. Simplify the recipes as needed.

★ Even if the person living with dementia can't help prepare food, he can still enjoy sitting in on the action and the conversation. Having the experience is more satisfying than sharing any dish of food.

Feed Friendships by Cooking

"Strange to see how a good dinner and feasting reconciles everybody." —Samuel Pepys

Nancy takes a deep breath as she let herself into her parents' house, trying to prepare herself. Lately, with her mom's dementia, the place has been an absolute mess. But today, the living room is surprisingly tidy.

"We're in the kitchen," her father calls. His voice sounds cheerful, and Nancy wonders what's going on; he's been so depressed lately.

Her mother sits at the table with their neighbor Pauline.

"Pauline came over, and we made lunch together," her father says. "Your mother made the egg salad sandwiches."

"Mom, you made the sandwiches?" Nancy asks. "I love your egg salad."

Her mother smiles.

"We used her old recipe card," Pauline says. "She did it all, including peeling the eggs."

As usual, Nancy has brought over a casserole for Sunday lunch, but she tucks it into the refrigerator and sits down to enjoy the meal, the first one her mother has prepared in ages.

After they eat, her father says solemnly, "There's more."

Pauline runs into the kitchen and brings out a plate with four cupcakes on it.

"Happy Birthday, darling," her father says.

Her mother smiles at her. Nancy wipes away a tear; she'd figured her parents were in too much chaos to remember her birthday. The cupcakes are piled with icing and over-decorated with sprinkles. They look absolutely delicious.

"Pauline helped with the cake mix, and your mother stirred in all the ingredients and decorated the cakes," her father says.

"Mom, this is wonderful," Nancy says. She hasn't seen her mom looking so happy and calm in ages.

"How old are you, dear?" her mother asks. Normally, that sort of remark makes Nancy want to curl into a little ball and cry, but today, she smiles as she says, "Forty-five, Mom." Then Nancy takes a big bite of cupcake and gives her mom a hug.

Sue (Suzanne) Fitzsimmons, MS, ARNP, has seen firsthand the power of purposeful cooking.

"Cooking is very personal, and it's central to a person's life," Sue says. "Many times, when people go deeper into dementia, they don't have the opportunity to prepare food. And they don't have a chance to make something for someone else."

Fixing a delicacy for someone else offers a tangible and delicious way to give back. Plus, it's something the care partner can brag about to family members and friends: "Your mom made a pie today." "Your father made us grilled cheese for lunch."

Here are a few easy cooking projects:

- **Butter Them Up**
  This is an example of "shake it until you make it." Put heavy cream in a container and shake until the fat separates from the buttermilk, leaving you with delicious butter. You

can involve multiple generations in this simple activity. Enhance the experience by adding music or sharing stories. Take turns shaking so no one gets too weary. Putting in a few marbles speeds up the process; just make sure you extract them before serving.

"Offering visitors a slice of banana bread with homemade butter is a great conversation starter," Sue says.

- **Well-Bread Lunches**
  Create sandwiches together for a simple and satisfying lunch. Consider peanut butter and jelly, cheese and pickles, or lunchmeat and tomatoes. If you want to get more complicated, make egg or tuna salad. You can always fancy up the meal by slicing the sandwich in quarters and adding decorative toothpicks.

- **Sampling S'mores**
  "Men often like to make s'mores," Sue says. Enjoy creating this campground favorite by stacking graham crackers, marshmallows, and chocolate and getting them all gooey and melted in the microwave. For additional flair, enjoy them in front of a fire or simulated fire.

- **Tea Times**
  One care partner team hosted a tea party for friends and family. They grew herbs and blended them into a unique tea. You can also buy herbs. For an easy tea bag, you can put the tea blend in a coffee filter and staple it together, or just buy bags at a teashop. To enhance the festive atmosphere, bake or decorate cookies.

Creative Sparks

★ Choose a time of day when everyone's rested and alert.

★ Go through favorite cookbooks or old recipe cards to discover a dish your partner might enjoy making.

★ Print out the recipe in large type, along with an ingredient and utensil list.

★ Make a shopping list and then go grocery shopping together. Put the list on a clipboard and, if appropriate, give your partner time to find each ingredient.

Build Brain Power with Culinary Creativity

"One cannot think well, love well, and sleep well, if one has not dined well." —Virginia Woolf

Rebecca Katz, author of *The Healthy Mind Cookbook*, sees food as a great equalizer, something anyone can enjoy regardless of abilities.

"It doesn't matter what you can remember," she says. "With cooking, you have to be in the present moment."

Even after Rebecca's father was diagnosed with dementia, he remained an appreciative and adventurous eater, and one of Rebecca's great joys was cooking for and with him.

She often invited her father to help her in the kitchen, and he liked tearing up herbs, adding ingredients into the pot, and stirring risotto, one of his favorite dishes. He then enjoyed sitting at the table, sharing the meal.

Fuel the Brain and Make Sense of the Senses

Even before she became a cookbook author, chef, and national speaker, Rebecca Katz loved spending time in the kitchen. She delighted in the flavors, textures, colors, and aromas of fruits and vegetables. And she was fascinated by fruits and vegetables that nourished body, mind, and spirit.

Rebecca focuses her nutritional choices on a "culinary pharmacy," an array of fruits, vegetables, herbs, and spices that affect the brain in positive ways. Her list includes lemons, oranges, mint, cashews, walnuts, olives, cinnamon, avocados, peaches, and kale. These super foods nurture and fuel the brain.

"Like many of us, people living with dementia have moods," Rebecca says. "If you offer them the right kinds of fuel, they may become happier and more engaged."

As people age, their sense of taste dims. Adding interesting spices and flavors sparks up the taste buds, spurs appetite, pleasurably engages the senses, and benefits the brain.

"When you cook familiar aromatic foods, such as onions, spaghetti, popcorn, chocolate, or spiced cider, the sense of smell can connect you to other memories," Rebecca says. "It's like listening to a piece of favorite music."

For a sensory, yet practical, culinary connection, Rebecca suggests recipes and experiences that involve texture, aroma, sight, and taste.

- Mix together whole pumpkin seeds, cashews, and walnuts for a healthful snack.
- Tear off mint leaves, slice citrus fruits, and put both in cool water for a flavorful, refreshing beverage.
- Strip kale off its thick stem and rip it into bite-size pieces. Store in a container until ready to prepare.
- Make hummus together by pouring cooked chickpeas in the blender and adding in lemon juice, tahini, and olive oil.
- Involve your partner in tasting and giving feedback. When a dish is nearly finished, offer a spoonful and ask, "On a scale of one to ten, how does this taste? What do you think it needs—more sweet, more salt, maybe a touch of lemon?"

Creative Sparks

★ Incorporate brain-boosting fruits and vegetables into your diet to improve health, disposition, and engagement.

★ Look for natural ways to spend time together in the kitchen. Add meal preparation into your weekly schedule, if possible.

★ When possible, engage all the senses during a cooking project.

★ Spice up your lives by adding in flavorful seasonings. Even spritzing on lemon juice or adding in cinnamon offers a pleasant zing.

A Feast for the Senses

"Good painting is like good cooking; it can be tasted, but not explained." —Maurice de Vlaminck

Judith Fertig's mom doesn't have dementia, but she can no longer cook. Still she loves vicariously feasting through reading the taste book she made for her daughters several decades ago. Many pages feature a family photo, a hand-written recipe, and an anecdote that brings the dishes to life. Judith's copy of this book is a family treasure.

Judith, a novelist and award-winning cookbook author, has created several taste books and understands what a meaningful and memorable gift they make. Inspired by her mom's book, Judith designed a "pie taste book" for her niece, a CPA who loves baking pies. A wedding present, her niece's book features cherished pie recipes, photos of relatives who helped bake them, two exotic crust recipes, and a picture of her niece's husband holding his favorites: sour cherry and key lime pie.

"Recipes are part of a family's legacy," Judith says. "It's fun to put together a taste book and discuss what you've already concocted and what dishes you might want to make."

Building a taste book can become a part of spending time together.

"During your visit, you can make a recipe, photograph the baking process and the finished dish, write down the story of the dish, and later add the finished page to the taste book," Judith suggests.

Invite friends and family to contribute, each sending a beloved recipe, a photo of the cook and the dish, and a story of preparing food or eating together. Those who like to eat but aren't much for hanging around the kitchen can design a taste book by going through old gourmet magazines and making collages of recipes and favorite dishes. Cutting and pasting is relaxing and offers time to discuss special meals and other food-related memories.

Taste books are conversation catalysts. When looking through them, add to the sensory experience by sharing aromatic herbs and spices, such as cinnamon, vanilla, and rosemary.

Creative Sparks

★ Select a theme that has meaning to your partner. Ideas could include Holiday Meals, Desserts, Birthday Parties, Cookies, or a specific era when she baked a lot.

★ Invite friends and family to contribute to the project.

★ Select recipes that are part of your family history.

★ Add photos and stories to heighten the experience.

★ Go online and design a taste book or use a scrapbook-type notebook or a photo album.

Nibble on a Few Extras

"A party without cake is just a meeting." —Julia Child

The Icing off the Cake

Decorating with icing can be enticing even for someone who isn't used to cooking. Buy or make icing, then decorate a plate, cupcake, or even a piece of toast using icing pens or making broad swoops with a knife.

A Recipe for Reminiscence

As her husband Charlie moved deeper into dementia, Elizabeth Miller bought a cookbook from his teenage years, the 1960s. They read through the recipes and highlighted the ones he remembered his mom making. Then, with Charlie as her sous-chef, Elizabeth made dishes such as chicken cacciatore, tuna casserole, and spaghetti and meatballs. They invited Charlie's childhood friends over for a meal and talked about old times while they chowed down on Johnny Marzetti Casserole, a fancy term for elbow macaroni and ground beef.

Favorite Foods and Taking the Stress out of Restaurants

Elizabeth and Charlie also made a scrapbook of Charlie's favorite foods, complete with photos, so Charlie can leaf through and remember what he likes to eat. When they plan to go out for dinner, they look at the book of favorites, and they review the menu online. Charlie decides what he'd like to eat before they go and he writes it down. That way, he's not overwhelmed in the restaurant.

Pizza Party

At Silverado/Memory Care Communities, people are often invited to build their own individual pizzas. Each person has a small round of dough, a dish of sauce to spread on it, an array of toppings to choose from, and some cheese to sprinkle on. The sensory taste-fest is fun for multi-generations and people of varying abilities, and it inspires a lot of conversation and decision-making.

Giving Bark

Stir purpose into the kitchen experience by baking dog biscuits for animals in a shelter.

CHAPTER SEVEN
Grow Together through Nature

Dig into Your Own Natural Resources

Snuggle Up with the Warm Puppy Solution

Connect with Chickens and Dogs and Llamas

Plant Tomatoes and Grow Relationships

Harvest Happiness through Volunteer Farming

Think Outside the House

Go Outdoors and Build Brain Health

Blossom with Flower Power

Dig into Your Own Natural Resources

"The greatest gift of the garden is the restoration
of the five senses." —Hanna Rion

"What does your mother like to do?" the nurse asks me. "Does she enjoy cooking, gardening, reading, movies?"

My mother, Fran, is a sweet little comma curled into a stern bracket of a wheelchair. She looks like someone who likes taking naps and staring into space. But the nurse is inviting me to see beyond this memory care community and tell her what brought my mother pleasure.

"Growing roses," I say, thinking of the fragrant Peace, Crimson Glory, and Tropicana roses in the yard of my growing up house in Memphis. "Looking at birds, taking walks, going swimming."

I dab at my eyes as I remember how beautifully my mom wove the outdoors into my life. And I renew my efforts to keep nature in her life by sitting with her in the sunny courtyard, visiting the elm and maples in front of the care facility, and bringing her small bouquets of roses, daisies, and lilies.

"Nature-oriented activities, such as growing and caring for plants, promote brain neuroplasticity and help us dream, experiment, learn, and create," says Garuth Chalfont, PhD, a leading practitioner in the art and science of healing gardens, therapeutic spaces, and dementia gardens, and author of the book *Dementia Green Care*.

This section blossoms with easy ideas for integrating the balm of animals, plants, and nature into your daily life. These creative experts will pique your curiosity with comfort chickens, fairy gardens, inland beaches, and yard tours.

"Nature-oriented activities, such as growing and caring for plants, promote brain neuroplasticity and help us dream, experiment, learn, and create."

Snuggle Up with the Warm Puppy Solution

"Happiness is a warm puppy." — Charles M. Schulz

"What am I supposed to do now?" Mollie asks. At age ninety-seven, her memory is fragmented, her speech repetitive. Her face, normally a canvas of beauty and repose, is drawn; her mouth is stretched thin and tight, and her eyes dart fearfully. "What I am supposed to do?"

My life partner Ron and I sit beside her on the sofa. Months earlier, she moved from her elegant, antique-laden apartment in a retirement community to a smaller venue on the assisted living floor.

"What would you like to do?" Ron, her son, says, touching Mollie's hand.

"I don't know. I want to die. I just want to die. What am I supposed to do?" Her rings clink as she clenches her hands. If she were steadier on her feet, she would pace, but she's too weak to do more than wobble down the hallway clinging to her walker.

"Mollie, would you like to listen to some music?" I ask. Over the weeks, Ron and I have struggled to find comforting and engaging words and activities. We've tried listening to music, singing, looking at nostalgic photos, bringing over old friends, reading poetry.

Though she enjoys moments of connection and respite, nothing seems to really soothe or please her. And nothing eases the gnawing agitation that stalks her waking hours. Except Lilly.

There's a knock on her door, and our friend Barb enters with Lilly close behind. Mollie smiles when she sees Lilly. She pats her leg, and Lilly leaps up, settling into Mollie's lap. Mollie pets the small, soft shih tzu and sighs. Her shoulders relax, and her eyes close. Lilly snuggles in and closes her eyes. The two sit silently, Mollie gently stroking Lilly. In one minute, Lilly accomplishes what Ron and I have been struggling to do for one hour: soothe and comfort Mollie.

Barb perches across from us on the edge of a recliner.

"We visited last week, and Mollie and Lilly just sat together for a long time," Barb tells us.

"I'm glad to see Lilly," Mollie says, still stroking the little dog.

"How've you been Mollie?" Barb asks.

"I went to Bingo," Mollie says.

We all grin. Mollie's prowess at games of chance remains legendary.

"Did you win?" I ask.

"Of course," Mollie says with a lilt in her voice.

Mollie talks and then dozes, while Lilly snoozes peacefully. Then Lilly stands, shakes herself, jumps down, and trots over to nuzzle Barb.

"I'll see you in a couple of days, Mollie," Barb tells her.

"Will you bring Lilly?" Mollie asks.

"Of course."

"I love that dog," Mollie says, closing her eyes, her face now serene.

We tiptoe out, leaving Mollie to her afternoon nap.

Connect with Chickens and Dogs and Llamas

"Animals are such agreeable friends— they ask no questions, they pass no criticisms." —George Eliot

It's Wednesday, and Travis is making his weekly visit to the memory care community. As he walks down the corridor into the common area, residents crowd around him, admiring him and petting him. Travis soaks up the attention while the residents revel in their visit with a real live llama.

Travis and his fellow llama Vijay live in a spacious pen just outside of LifeCare Center of Nashoba Valley in Littleton, Massachusetts. Their companions include five goats and an alpaca named Medi (short for Medi Care). Community members can stroll around and observe the animals from a paved walkway or a nearby bench. The area is a favorite destination for visitors and residents, offering natural entertainment and an easy topic of conversation.

Observe Those Birds of a Feather

"Our director understands how beneficial animals can be," says Lauren Gaffney, Memory Support Unit Program Director. "We're all encouraged to bring in our pets, and we also have volunteers who bring their pets to visit."

"Having the animals to watch is like the best TV program ever."

The Memory Care Unit has its own trio of busy hens that the residents have named Elsie, Mae Belle, and Beulah. The chickens live in a pen right outside an observation window in the courtyard. Residents flock to watch the creatures; staff members often hold one of the birds so residents and families can savor petting their soft feathers. Even when there's not a direct interaction, studies have observed that being around animals reduces anxiety.

"The chickens always offer us something new," Lauren says. "Our activities person gathers eggs, and we examine them and talk about egg experiences and memories. Having the animals to watch is like the best TV program ever."

Rescue a Dog and Revitalize Conversations

When they're not patting llamas and observing chickens, the memory care residents look after Lucy, their rescue greyhound. Lucy is recovering from a difficult life, and the home's gentle touch and companionable environment is helping her learn to trust again.

On a quiet morning, a group may circle around Lucy and watch her sleep.

"Isn't she lovely?" one says.

"She seems to be getting calmer."

"I have a treat for her later."

Lucy stimulates conversation, increases social connections, and brings out people's nurturing instincts: they love to pet and brush her.

The Two-L Llama Is a Catalyst

The animals have helped in other ways. Marie, a new resident, was having trouble standing up from a sitting position; she was afraid she'd fall if she leaned forward. She'd been to physical therapy, and staff had worked with her, yet her fear persisted. But when Travis walked into the room, Marie instantly leaned forward to pet the llama.

> "I firmly believe that animals are integral in encouraging interactions and reducing agitation. Plus, they're delightful to have around."

"The llama opened a door for her," Lauren says.

The animals help the staff as well, giving them a chance to de-stress during their day.

"I firmly believe that animals are integral in encouraging interactions and reducing agitation," says Lauren. "Plus, they're delightful to have around."

Creative Sparks

★ If you have pets, invite your partner to stay involved, brushing, petting, feeding, or playing with them.

★ Use animals as conversation catalysts. Some friends and family may feel awkward visiting; having a pet along offers an icebreaker and invites reminiscence.

★ If you don't have animals, encourage friends and family to bring well-behaved pets to visit at home or in the care center.

★ Take a trip to a pet shop, animal shelter, or a petting
zoo. Some zoos have special programs for people living
with dementia and their care partners. Others have
an outreach program and will bring an assortment of
creatures to a care facility or community center.

Plant Tomatoes and Grow Relationships

"Gardening is cheaper than therapy and you
get tomatoes." —Author Unknown

"Mable, I could use your assistance this morning," Lori Condict
says. "The tomatoes are ripe, and I need help picking them. Are
you available?"

Mable nods. Lori waits while Mable puts on her gardening
hat and gloves. Then they join others from the memory care
community outside in the garden.

"What are you thinking about Mable?" Lori asks, handing her
a small bucket.

"My first bite of summer tomato."

"Let's try one of these," Lori says. She knows that Mable and
her husband used to have a vast vegetable and flower plot.

Mable plucks a cherry tomato off the vine and pops it into
her mouth.

Slowly, she picks another and plops it in her bucket. Others in
her community are also harvesting the tomatoes.

"We'll be sharing our vegetables with the food bank, so others less fortunate will enjoy this fresh produce," Lori reminds her.

"That's good," Mable says. "Everyone needs to taste these tomatoes."

Mable lives in the memory care unit in Chestnut Glen Assisted Living by Americare in St. Peters, Missouri. She is one of the fifteen residents working on the Operation Riverfront gardening project. Lori, the activities director in the care facility, is a city girl. But she wasn't bothered by her lack of experience; she knew she'd have plenty of help from her residents. She also knew they would thrive knowing they had a purpose and were giving back to their community.

Seeding Empowerment

Lori started simply with a bunch of tomato, cucumber, squash, peppers, and pea seeds—pretty and colorful vegetables that would remind residents of their home gardens. Lori had tasks for all abilities: some held little containers while another filled them with dirt; some tamped in the seeds, and others labeled them. Lori provided everyone with special hats and gloves.

"Growing vegetables reminds them they are still valuable, and we need their talents and skills."

While they worked, they reminisced.

"Did you ever grow tomatoes?" Lori asked.

"Oh yes," one woman answered. "My son Jack watered them every night."

"My son liked to weed," said another.

They talked about their favorite tomato dishes and discussed summertime activities and more.

Every evening the group watered, each person holding a small container of water.

"Who cares if it takes twenty minutes to water one plant," Lori says, "or five minutes to pick one bean. Growing vegetables reminds them they are still valuable, and we need their talents and skills."

Sharing the Bounty

> "People who'd been depressed and disengaged got involved."

When it was time to share with the local food pantry, the residents did the harvesting and packing. One resident, a former social worker who was going through a difficult time emotionally, cheered up when Lori asked her to keep track of how much they gave away.

"We had planters, pickers, packers, counters, and a watering crew," Lori says. "People who'd been depressed and disengaged got involved. Through working on the project, they felt alive and useful; they had a purpose."

Lori constantly explores ways to keep her gardeners growing. During the holiday season, they operated a food drive for other seniors. They sorted the donated food, counted it, and packed it.

Lori is planning a project that would benefit a local hospital.

"You take away their car, their spouse, their house, their job—you have to give them back a purpose," Lori believes.

One tomato plant at a time, these residents are growing their skills, nourishing their souls, and feeding their community.

Creative Sparks

★ Select flowers, plants, vegetables, and herbs that are pretty, colorful, easy to grow, and have some meaning to the person living with dementia.

★ Create small tasks that are interesting and pleasurable.

★ To increase the sense of purpose, find ways to share blooms, cuttings, vegetables, and herbs with family, friends, and community members.

★ For those who can't go outdoors, bring the plants to them in containers.

★ Infuse the work with opportunities for conversation.

Harvest Happiness through Volunteer Farming

"To forget how to dig the earth and to tend the soil is to forget ourselves." —Mahatma Gandhi

Seattle's Rainier Beach Urban Farm and Wetlands is abuzz with volunteers. Some sit in the greenhouse, pressing seeds into rich, moist potting soil. Some fill up watering cans and others walk amongst the tomatoes and peppers, carefully pouring the water. Others weed or harvest tender lettuce. Some gardeners work independently while a support person gently guides others. The volunteers represent diversity in ages, ethnicities, and abilities, including East African elders from the community and people living with dementia.

"It's so peaceful I want to live here," Helen says, as a bald eagle soars overhead. As a younger woman, she'd cherished her time in the garden. Since she was diagnosed with dementia, her time in nature has been limited. For Helen, this experience feels like coming home.

"Many of our volunteers are living with dementia," says Tamara Keefe, one of the organization's representatives involved in supporting the dementia-friendly urban farm experience. "They enjoy the gardening projects, but they also like talking, working together, and spending meaningful time together."

Part of the Friday morning experience is eating a delicious lunch cooked by individuals from the East African community and supplemented with produce from the garden. After working hard in the morning, sharing a meal cements the sense of community. There are communication barriers, but one of the volunteers suggested, "We aren't going to learn each other's languages, but I wonder if we can sing together."

"The idea of singing together, coming from a participant with memory loss, opened up everyone's world," Tamara says.

Gradually, over the months, the various volunteers have come to feel connected, circumventing the language barriers through smiling and gesturing.

Contribute to the Community

"A dementia diagnosis does not need to be the end of enjoying life, pursuing interests, or contributing to one's community. Volunteer opportunities can open doors and allow people to continue to grow."

Working at the farm gives people with dementia a chance to give back, take a break from their ordinary routines, enjoy the natural surroundings, do something meaningful with their care partner, and meet new people. Plus, they share a good meal with fascinating folks.

"A dementia diagnosis does not need to be the end of enjoying life, pursuing interests, or contributing to one's community," Tamara says. "Volunteer opportunities can open doors and allow people to continue to grow."

Creative Sparks

★ When gardening together, invite your partner to choose the tasks she'll most enjoy.

★ Enjoy talking or singing while you work.

★ Offer a multisensory experience by watering, planting, weeding, and harvesting.

★ When possible, taste the harvest. After your hard work, share a snack or a meal that includes something from the garden.

Think Outside the House

"I go to nature to be soothed and healed, and to
have my senses put in order." —John Burroughs

"Shall we spend the afternoon at the beach?" Harry asks his
wife, Madeline.

A smile lights her face, and she nods. It's a gloomy day in
Yorkshire, England, and Madeline has been staring outside all
morning. Harry can feel her restlessness.

"Let's bring a picnic," Harry says.

"Lemonade," Madeline says.

"Yes. Do you want cheese or tuna fish sandwiches?"

"Cheese."

"Without spending a lot of money, you can fashion an amazing atmosphere in a small space."

Together they go into the kitchen, and Harry makes their lunch. Then he packs a hamper and leads Madeline to their screened-in porch. The deck chairs are waiting. A bright beach umbrella leans against the wall. He turns on the CD player, and the soothing sound of rolling ocean waves blends in with backyard birdsong. He rubs a little sunscreen on Madeline's hands, the kind she used when they were dating so many years ago. He helps her take off her shoes and pushes over a container of sand. It's warm and dry, and Madeline wiggles her toes in it. Though they are miles from the seashore, by using creativity and imagination, they still enjoy the feeling of being at the beach.

"Without spending a lot of money, you can fashion an amazing atmosphere in a small space," says Claire Craig, PhD, coauthor of *Creativity and Communication in Persons with Dementia: A Practical Guide*. "There are no limits: I've seen indoor jungles, beaches, formal plantings, and forests."

For inspiration, Claire attends flower and water garden shows and visits websites.

Nurture with Nature

"People with dementia often feel a sense of calm and connectedness when they're outdoors," says Claire. "When people are not grounded in their natural surroundings, they can feel disoriented and confused."

Claire sees the outdoors as a place to unite art and nature. Many people relate to the seasons through gardening, farming, and lawn care. Many relish walking or sitting outside, feeling the fresh air, seeing majestic oaks or fragrant pines, breathing in just-bloomed lilacs and crimson roses, watching squirrels, and hearing lyrical birdsong.

"Look at your outdoor space as an opportunity," Claire advises. "Ask yourself, 'How can we make this space our own?' Think of projects you can do as a team. Consider building something simple out of wood. Glue it together if you don't want to use nails. Decorate planters with paints or paste-on shells, tiles, pebbles, mosaic pieces, and more."

"People with dementia often feel a sense of calm and connectedness when they're outdoors."

Poetry rocks, literally. Claire guides people in gluing short poems, inspirational sayings, or copies of favorite photos onto smooth rocks, and then varnishing them. They will fade with the weather but make lovely gifts or garden accents. She also suggests painting rocks. To create a spontaneous outdoor art gallery, she pins copies of photos on a clothesline and discusses them as they flap in the breeze.

Creative Sparks

★ Think of simple ways to weave nature-related experiences into your day. Include walking, picnicking, gardening, and creating outdoor art. For indoor or outdoor connections, try photography along with bird, animal, and people watching.

★ Take an indoor activity outside. Knit, draw, or put together puzzles. Go to a nearby park and listen to music.

★ Spread a bright cloth on a table, the ground, or across your lap for an instant picnic. Enjoy your traditional fare and add lively music or outdoor sounds, using a soundtrack of fireworks, train whistles, and running, laughing children.

★ Make a list of favorite outdoor venues for both yourself and your partner.

★ Focus on the components of the outdoors experience that were most important for your partner. Did he love to pack the lunch and organize the maps? Was putting on a backpack and hat important? Did he especially enjoy the car or train ride there? Did he revel in the sounds of the woodlands? Once you've answered these questions, experiment with ways to recreate those evocative and comforting outdoor atmospheres.

Go Outdoors and Build Brain Health

"An early morning walk is a blessing for the whole day."—Henry David Thoreau

As soon as Fred starts pacing, Helen invites him outside for a walk. She's mapped out a perfect ten-minute stroll in their English village, complete with interesting sights. Sometimes she asks their neighbor's standard poodle to join them. People always stop and talk to the dog, and Helen and Fred relish the extra conversations. But today, it's just the two of them, walking to the corner where they admire the neighbor's fieldstone wall that Fred helped build. They look at the crabapple tree that arches over the sidewalk. In season, crabapples spill everywhere. Talking about crabapples can make Fred hungry for Helen's apple pie, which they've taken to making together. They hold hands and head to the small playground with one slide and three swings. They sit on an old wooden bench and watch children playing. On the way home, they discuss the flowers they see. The short walk is a respite for both of them, offering fresh air, sunshine, a sense of serenity, and a connection with each other and the outdoors.

"Research shows that nature-based activity is therapeutic and is essentially a form of treatment for dementia symptoms, helping a person remain at home longer," says Garuth Chalfont, PhD, a member of American Society of Landscape Architects and author of the *Dementia Green Care Handbook*. Garuth is internationally known for his work in designing, building, and researching gardens that benefit people with dementia. He also partners with care facilities and families, helping them integrate nature into their living quarters and their outdoors.

Gathering flowers, walking down a tree-lined sidewalk, plucking a cherry tomato off its vine, watering a house plant, gazing out the window at chickadees—these meaningful natural activities increase pleasure, relaxation, social interactions, and sensory stimulation.

"Research shows that nature-based activity is therapeutic and is essentially a form of treatment for dementia symptoms, helping a person remain at home longer.

Smorgasbord Your Yard

"Enjoying the garden goes beyond just walking around," Garuth says.

Whether you have an acre, a few hundred feet, or a couple of indoor containers, consider making a smorgasbord out of your yard by adding taste, aroma, and touch to your garden. What can you literally go out and eat? What can you cut and bring in for drawing, making crafts, or admiring? Does your partner have a favorite plant or a flower that reminds him of earlier times? Is there a color or scent that excites him?

Think of Views That Wow

Imagine you're hosting a guided tour of your yard. What is the most thrilling part of your lawn? A blooming rose bush? A bird bath? A wise old fir tree?

"By creating a tour, you're taking a new look at your environment. You're telling a story and engaging your partner," Garuth says.

Stir up conversation by focusing on one area at a time. Perhaps discuss the hanging bird feeder. Or a seashell you two found on your last vacation. Then observe the birdbath or other water feature. Do you have a bench? Sit down and talk about what you see. Create a "wow" ending with something that is fun and dramatic, such as a ceramic gnome peeking from behind a rock, a modest flock of pink plastic flamingos hiding behind the hydrangeas, or a bright sculpted yellow sun affixed to the front door.

Seeing your yard as a living story may inspire you to add in a playful spinner, a cute stone animal, or a beautiful rock. Vary the environment throughout the year. String fairy lights and add flickering yard ornaments in winter. In spring, drape colorful yarn over branches for birds to weave into their nests.

See Nature from the Inside Out

"Look at that yellow finch," Mary says, handing the binoculars to her husband Joe. Joe's hands wobble as he adjusts the view.

"There are two of them. Probably flown in from up north on their way to warm weather," he says. "And there's a brown bird beside them." He pours himself a little more coffee from the thermos.

Mary opens their bird book.

"Seems like some kind of sparrow," she says. She passes the book to Joe.

"Any yard, garden, balcony, or other outdoor
space can offer familiar sensations, while also
stimulating the heart, mind, and spirit."

For years, the two of them were avid bird watchers. In earlier times, they would have had this conversation hunched in a bird blind or standing in tall woods, peering up into dense foliage. But they're now watching the woodpeckers, chickadees, and finches from the comfort of their living room, listening to a CD of bird songs. When Joe's dementia progressed and he could no longer enjoy the rigors of hiking and standing, they rearranged their living room furniture, so they could sit facing the front lawn. They installed bird feeders and a birdbath and continued their hobby.

"Any yard, garden, balcony, or other outdoor space can offer familiar sensations, while also stimulating the heart, mind, and spirit," Garuth says. "Look around your living quarters and ask, 'Where are the best outdoor views? Where is the most sunlight?' You may need to cut down a light-blocking bush or move a sofa, but you will discover areas where you and your partner can enjoy sitting and watching nature."

Green Up Your House

The table is strewn with greenery, acorns, sticks, and pinecones. The residents gently finger strands of ivy and brilliant orange maple leaves. One person examines a plump pinecone, and another rubs sage between her fingers, releasing its fragrance.

"Touching natural objects awakens the senses."

Garuth encourages people to connect with the natural world by gathering objects, such as nuts, berries, sprigs, rocks, and flowers, and then drawing pictures of them.

"Touching natural objects awakens the senses," Garuth says. "Drawing plants can be very therapeutic, offering a meditative and peaceful experience."

"Art can keep the conversation going in lieu of words."

Garuth believes drawing to communicate is a basic human ability, used since earliest times to make sense of the world.

"It is especially important to develop an affinity for drawing before verbal abilities fail," Garuth says. "Art can keep the conversation going in lieu of words."

Feed Your Creative Spirit and Your Wildlife

Garuth sees the activity of feeding creatures as a multifaceted circle. You may scavenge green apples or crabapples that have fallen from nearby trees. You can string these edibles, cranberries, or popcorn, using a dull darning needle, and set them outside to attract wildlife.

"You gather the substances, make the craft, return it to the garden, and then watch the animals' response," Garuth says. "That enriches the natural connection and engages you in the complete cycle."

Pot Seeds and Design a Fairy Garden

For a relaxing experience, gather potting soil, water, and green bean seeds. Spoon the soil into small pots or into an empty egg carton. Place one seed in each pot and cover with soil, then pour in a little water. Don't worry about outcome; just enjoy the experience. Let your partner lead the activity; he may end up drawing with his finger in the dirt or forming mud pies.

"Touching soil and planting may trigger memories and ideas from earlier years," Garuth says.

Create a miniature world with an indoor fairy garden. An old container provides the ideal setting for soil, moss, a few micro plants, miniscule ceramic animals, and a tiny table and chairs. Collect small sticks, leaves, rocks, and shells to add to the fairy kingdom. You can build a pebble pathway or create furniture out of bendable twigs and grasses. You and your partner can enjoy rearranging the décor and adding little extras, making this project imaginative and interactive.

Creative Sparks

★ Seek ways to incorporate nature into your life, both indoors and outdoors.

★ Create observation spots in your living space so you can enjoy looking outdoors. Even watching the weather helps people feel engaged in the natural environment.

★ Improve your view with interesting additions, such as bird feeders and birdhouses, bubbling fountains, wind chimes, wind spinners, outdoor sculpture, and various plants and herbs.

★ Add resilient plants to your home.

★ Bring in natural objects to touch, identify, arrange, and draw.

★ Create miniature fairy gardens.

★ When possible, grow vegetables and other edibles, as well as using favorite flowers and plants.

★ Map out a walking tour of your yard so you have several interesting destinations to discuss and explore. This can be as simple as an old pair of work boots with the toes cut out for sedum to grow. Hang ceramic animal sculptures on trees or against the house for additional accents.

- ★ Design a ten-minute walk with plenty of sensory stimulation. If needed, include a resting place along the route.

- ★ Visit garden centers, parks, playgrounds, and zoos for a rich natural experience.

- ★ Increase your popularity by taking a dog with you on a walk, either your own or borrow your neighbor's pup.

Blossom with Flower Power

"Deep in their roots, all flowers keep
the light." —Theodore Roethke

Martha's hands shake as she pours water into a small vase. She stares at a pile of flowers on the green cutting board and fingers a daisy. In earlier times, in addition to working as a schoolteacher, she was a master gardener with a lavish wildflower plot. But since she's moved into a memory care community, she's shied away from gardening activities; the dirt seems to bother her.

Now Martha lifts the daisy and puts it in the vase. It's too tall, and she pulls it out, takes a small pair of safety scissors, and cuts off part of the stem, just so. She selects a yellow chrysanthemum, then adds a red rose and a spray of delicate white baby's breath. Martha turns the vase around, surveying it from all angles, and smiles.

Tom and Karen Brenner discuss this and other Montessori-oriented activities in their book *You Say Goodbye and We Say Hello: The Montessori Method for Positive Dementia Care.*

Trigger Muscle Memory

Combining Tom's background in gerontology and Karen's career as a Montessori teacher, they help families and facilities identify projects and activities that speak to the individual living with dementia.

"Letting people work with meaningful objects plays to their strengths and invites muscle memory," Tom says.

Muscle memory is responsible for activities such as walking, talking, and riding a bike. In a 1997 study of people living with Alzheimer's, researchers found that muscle memory functions longer than other types of memory.

Montessori encouraged natural materials whenever possible. For a gardener like Martha, the smell and feel of the flowers can evoke many muscle memories. Pouring water, placing blooms, and cutting stems engage motor skills, range of motion, and sense of aesthetics.

"This simple activity allows Martha to add beauty to her environment," Karen says. "But you don't have to be a gardener to enjoy being involved with flowers."

Hold onto Natural Objects

Flower arranging lends itself to teamwork and conversation. If your partner is overwhelmed by too many steps, she can pour water into vases and select a single blossom. You can

> "It's important to put something meaningful in people's hands."

discuss where the bloom goes in the arrangement. Enrich or alter the experience by adding different kinds of greenery. You can create a wreath or a centerpiece by working with pinecones, acorns, pine boughs, prairie grasses, and dried berries.

"It's important to put something meaningful in people's hands," Tom says. This can include brightly colored autumn leaves, dried out brown leaves, snow, mud, sand, and sticks.

Creative Sparks

★ Collect flowers and greenery from your garden or buy an inexpensive assortment from the grocery store.

★ Lay out the blooms and other natural objects on a table, along with safety scissors, a small pitcher of water, and several vases.

★ Discuss the blossoms, focusing on open-ended, failure-free questions, such as, "Which of the flowers do you like best? What do you like about them?"

★ Talk about how many arrangements you'd like to make.

★ Invite your partner to take the lead, helping only as needed.

★ Enjoy and appreciate your partner's efforts with affirming, observational comments, such as, "I really like the way you put the gold and red mum together with the pine bough." Or, "That ivy adds a lot to the red roses."

★ Display the arrangements so you and guests can enjoy them.

★ Add extra meaning to the activity by making a special flower display for a friend or relative.

CHAPTER EIGHT

Engage Imagination with Movies, Puppets, Clowns, and a Dash of Drama

Fan Your Imagination

Treat Yourselves to a Reel Boost

Give a Hand with Puppets

Clown Around for Connection

Ignite Your Creativity

Fan Your Imagination

"The possible's slow fuse is lit by the imagination." —Emily Dickinson

During her time in the memory care community, my mother fell in love with a baby doll. She held the doll, rocked her, talked to her, and connected with her in a pure and stress-free way. While I was searching my mother's face to see if she remembered me, the baby doll was sweetly lying still in her arms, not expecting a thing.

Karrie Marshall, author of *Puppetry in Dementia Care: Connecting through Creativity and Joy*, says, "When I first introduced puppetry into adult care work, there was a hesitant response. But puppetry has a long history with adults, making social and political comment. There is also a magical quality to puppets. They engage with emotions that go beyond words or memory." Karrie's book is filled with stories that show how people with dementia focus on the puppet and completely ignore the puppeteers, the staff, and the relatives.

Mom didn't get to meet any puppets or clowns during those days, but if she had, I'm sure she would have loved them as well. They, too, offer a stress-free connection for the person living with dementia. The experts in this chapter offer easy ways to honor imagination and invite therapeutic connections through those whimsical creatures and through playful brainstorming sessions, movies, and more.

Treat Yourself to a Reel Boost

"Cinema can fill in the empty spaces of your life
and your loneliness."—Pedro Almodóvar

The Coolidge Corner Theater in Brookline, Massachusetts, is packed with moviegoers, munching popcorn and talking animatedly. Today instead of trailers announcing upcoming films, there is a playful game inviting people to listen to a few clues, then guess what movie clips they will be watching.

"A love story featuring farmers, ranchers, horses, and cows," has people calling out *Oklahoma*. Soon viewers are watching an opening segment of this legendary 1950s film: a handsome cowboy riding his horse slowly through a cornfield and singing "Oh What a Beautiful Mornin'."

After an eight-minute segment, the moderator returns to stir up a discussion about what they've seen.

"What's the most beautiful thing you've ever experienced?" he asks.

"The first time I saw my granddaughter," someone says.

Another says, "A sunset."

Some of them talk about seeing this film in their younger years. After a good conversation, the moderator tosses out a few hints about the next film clip, and the process continues until all eight film segments are watched and discussed.

Meet Me at the Movies

This film series, *Meet Me at the Movies,* is for people living with dementia and their care partners. John Zeisel, who masterminded the renowned Meet Me at MoMA (Museum of Modern Art) program with his collaborator Sean Caulfield, created a template that features eight engaging clips from classic films with iconic actors and emotional themes. The segments are five to eight minutes long. Four of the films feature music; two are comedies, and two are dramas. Between each segment, a moderator orchestrates an open-ended conversation.

"During the movie watching, the four 'A's of Alzheimer's'—aggression, anxiety, agitation, and apathy—melt away."

"Movies are a big part of my life," one participant says. "This event brought tears to my eyes." Another woman adds, "Nothing works better than grabbing people's attention from a dramatic perspective."

"During the movie watching, the four 'A's of Alzheimer's'—aggression, anxiety, agitation, and apathy—melt away," John says. "Husbands and wives who walk in feeling tense are soon relaxing, holding hands like they did when they first met, and laughing in the dark theater."

Creating a Meaningful Movie Experience

Vicki Stoecklin created her own cinema program, one that fit her needs as a woman living with early onset dementia.

"After I lost track of the plot during several movie watching sessions, my husband asked if he should stop every ten or fifteen minutes and talk about what we'd seen," Vicki says. "I loved the idea. Our interaction allowed me to relax while I was watching, knowing he would soon clear up any confusion."

Family members can easily design their own home theater experience. John suggests making the evening engaging, social, and entertaining. Select films that evoke a variety of emotions and invite discussion.

For shorter segments, turn to YouTube or select scenes from favorite DVDs. You can also enjoy watching classic TV programs, such as *I Love Lucy*. At appropriate points, pause the video for conversation. Ask for impressions and any thoughts. Add your own observations.

Creative Sparks

★ Select treasured scenes from a favorite full-length film or watch the entire film depending on timing and attention span. Use the closed caption option if hearing is an issue.

★ In selecting scenes, look for five-minute episodes that include a whole mini-story with a beginning, middle, and end—such as the classic *I Love Lucy* chocolate factory scene.

★ Before watching, prepare your usual movie snacks.

★ Talk about the film in advance, discussing the plot, the actors, and any memories you might have of the show.

★ Take breaks as often as you like to talk about the film and refresh snacks. When attention lags, stop watching.

★ Invite others to join you. A film can bridge generations, giving parents, children, and grandchildren something to share.

★ Some recommended films include *The Wizard of Oz, Oklahoma, Camelot, Guys and Dolls, It's a Wonderful Life, Casablanca, The Glenn Miller Story, Sound of Music, Singin' in the Rain, The Princess Bride, The Graduate.*

★ Select classic TV shows that interest your partner, such as *The Honeymooners.* Other recommended shows include *The Andy Griffith Show, Bonanza, The Carol Burnett Show, The Lawrence Welk Show,* and *Leave it to Beaver.*

Give a Hand with Puppets

"There are many advantages in puppets. They never argue and they have no private lives." —Oscar Wilde

Veronica Kaninska puts her bag of puppets on a table in the care home's community area and instantly Gerda, one of the elders, comes over and touches a bright yellow monkey puppet. Veronica takes the puppet, opens its mouth, and says, "Hello," in a high monkey-like voice.

"Hello," Gerda answers.

"How are you today?" the monkey asks.

Gerda touches its smiling face. "Aren't you supposed to be in the zoo?" she says.

Gerda is often silent and non-communicative, but she's relaxed and outgoing with the puppet.

"Puppets can be an imaginative and powerful tool for connecting with people living with dementia," Veronica says.

Puppets are only one of Veronica's many artistic interests and talents. Born in the Ukraine, she studied puppetry, theatrical arts, and opera before moving to the United States and settling in Brooklyn, New York. She intended to pursue an operatic career, but a temporary job as a recreation therapist working with elders turned into a full-time passion.

Offer a Puppet Rx

"Puppetry is an ancient art form, and people often see puppets as being safe to talk to," Veronica says. "Plus a puppet can say things that real people can't."

One of Veronica's puppets is Dr. Moody, who checks on moods. He still makes house calls, and he's especially helpful with those who struggle with behavioral issues.

"How are you?" Dr. Moody asks Ralph, a memory care elder who is having a very bad day.

"Terrible," Ralph says.

"I have a prescription for you," Dr. Moody announces.

Ralph leans forward, ready to hear this odd, little doctor's idea.

"I want you to laugh out loud three times a day."

Ralph laughs; the puppet prescription is already working.

Coax Out Personal Stories

Veronica uses puppets with groups and individuals.

"Puppets can reach people who are not very active," Veronica says. "They're visual, three-dimensional, and people can touch them."

One of Veronica's clients was nonverbal. Veronica visited her, showing her a green Elmo-like puppet and letting the puppet do the talking. But after several visits, the client still hadn't responded.

"I was about to give up when she started to copy the puppet's movement," Veronica says. "The puppet moved his hands left and right, and she mimicked the motion. The puppet blew a kiss, and she blew a kiss to the puppet. This was a breakthrough."

"Puppets can reach people who are not very active."

Puppets talk to everyone and can often coax out stories. For weeks Veronica had tried to engage Beth in the puppet group activities. Beth was sweet and quiet, wandering around and not sticking with the group. Then the puppet asked about her family.

Veronica was surprised when Beth answered, "Once I had a son, and he died and everything got screwed up."

"We didn't even know she'd had a son," Veronica says. "Beth had been silently grieving, and no one knew. She told the puppet, not me."

Use Puppets in Various Venues

Puppets are multitalented and can work in physical, cognitive, social, emotional, and spiritual domains. A stick puppet can play ball or toss a balloon. Most puppets can sing. All puppets that work in therapeutic settings are good listeners.

You don't need to be a puppeteer or have a talent for voiceovers to bring a puppet to life.

Creative Sparks

★ Buy or make a simple sock puppet. Choose a puppet your partner can relate to. For dog lovers, try a puppy puppet. Some women may relate to a grandmother figure. Make sure your puppet is friendly and has a great sense of humor.

★ Talk to your partner using the puppet's voice. Once you start talking, the puppet will guide you, even if you think you don't know what to do.

★ If you don't want to talk, put on music and let the puppet move to the rhythm. You're still capturing attention.

★ If your partner doesn't respond, try different things. The puppet can sing a favorite song, tell a joke, move around in a playful way, and ask a question.

Clown Around for Connection

"A clown is like aspirin, only he works twice as fast." —Groucho Marx

"Once we put on our noses, there's no confusing us with healthcare staff or social workers," says Magdalena Schamberger of Edinburgh, Scotland.

The red noses signify that Magdalena and her extended "clown family" are part of Hearts & Minds Elderflowers Programme. The performers in this unique program dance, sashay, stride, and tiptoe into healthcare facilities and residential homes, sparking creative, playful, and meaningful communication and engagement with the community members.

Each performer has a special name and a unique history. Mitzi Elderflower, Magdalena's clown persona, is a cousin from Austria who came to Edinburgh for a weekend visit. She liked the city so much, she never left. Her relatives include Spud, Handsome, Honeybunch, Sweetie Pie, and Pickle.

"Clowns have a positive outlook. They're trained to leave quiet space so people with dementia can initiate and contribute ideas."

Magdalena serves as Cofounder and Artistic Director of Hearts & Minds and has international experience performing, directing, and researching in the field of performing arts and dementia. Although the Elderflower family is comprised of professional performers trained to work with people living with dementia, Magdalena believes family care partners can easily work with some of the basic clowning concepts.

"Clowns have a positive outlook. They're trained to leave quiet space so people with dementia can initiate and contribute ideas," Magdalena says.

Red Noses Rule

On one of his weekly visits to a care home, Handsome might stride in, wiggle his red nose, tweak his black bow tie, and strike a chord on his ukulele to create interest. His clown sister Sweetie Pie wobbles right beside him, sporting a lime-green hair bow and pink barrettes that complement her ruby nose.

"We have a cousin who came to visit for two days, and four years later, she's still here," Spud might say to the residents with extreme mock seriousness. "Whatever shall we do? What would you do?"

"Change the locks," one woman says.

"But she cooks dinner for us every Tuesday," Sweetie Pie says. "And she bakes a delicious apple cake."

"Make the best of it," another resident advises.

"The community members here are surrounded with competent people meeting their care needs," says Magdalena. "Elderflowers treat these residents like experts and give them a chance to offer advice."

The Elderflowers frequently ask residents to help them make choices.

"Shall I wear my blue dancing slippers or my red tennis shoes when I go to the wedding?" Pickle might ask. For people with low verbal skills, Pickle will hold up each pair of shoes and give them time to choose. For a more verbal person, she'll pause, waiting to hear the shoe color. It's all in good fun, and the residents come to life, enjoying a chance to laugh and pretend.

Swearing by Clown Power

Sometimes, clowns can serve as relief valves. One resident, Alan, struggled with anger issues and lashed out occasionally. Magdalena was standing near Alan, dressed as Mitzi, her clown persona, when Alan started clutching his fist and swearing. Mitzi held playful eye contact with him and blurted out a made-up swear word. Alan stared at her. Then he smiled and began to make up cuss words as well. The clown had diffused a tense situation.

> Clowns also lift people out of their ordinary lives.

"I may hold an umbrella over our heads to create a little private space," Magdalena says. "Sometimes I spread a blanket over a sofa to simulate a picnic area." She may invite residents to pretend they're at a tea plantation or mention that Monday is Blue Day or Sunshine Day. Her goal is to circumvent their routine and stimulate the brain.

"People switch off during the ordinary," Magdalena says.

"I may hold an umbrella over our heads
to create a little private space."

Join the Red Nose Appreciation Society

The Elderflowers are professional performers and are trained in the art of clowning and in wearing the red nose to make those connections. The color red draws people's attention and helps those with vision problems access your eyes and face.

The red nose also gives permission to play.

"Even if you are not trained in clowning, this invitation to play may be achieved in other ways," Magdalena advises.

Experiment with props, such as hats, cameras, and maps. Put on a top hat, then hand it over and let your partner try it on. Take turns with dress-up objects.

"We're trying to create a sense of home and belonging," Magdalena says. "The Elderflowers welcome all into their circle."

Creative Sparks

★ Be curious.

★ Adopt a positive attitude and say yes to everything your partner proposes.

★ Concoct a costume that indicates playfulness. This can be an unusual hat, a funny sweater, or mismatched socks.

★ Ask for advice on a pretend problem. Offer two choices and enough time to make a comment or decision. Enthusiastically embrace the suggestions.

★ Share a basket of props, such as ties, beads, and scarves. Try on different items together and talk about how each makes you feel.

★ Zoom past ordinary life by putting a magical spin on the day. Propose an impromptu tea party or announce that it's National Exotic Tea day.

★ Fail cheerfully.

Ignite Your Creativity

"Imagination is the highest kite
one can fly." —Author Unknown

At first, I think Debra Campbell is wasting her time. She kneels in front of a gentleman who appears to be asleep. She holds up a vacuum cleaner tube and asks again, "Devin, what else could we use this for, besides cleaning the rug?"

Next to me, Marilyn, a lovely woman with beautifully coiffed silver hair and a coral necklace that matches her shirt, whispers, "Devin may have something up his sleeve." Marilyn lives in this memory care community and has already given me the inside scoop on several of the other residents.

Still, Devin does not stir, but Debra does not deter. She remains patient, alert to the possibilities of hidden treasures just waiting to be unearthed.

Debra is Executive Director of Kansas City Senior Theatre. Thirty minutes ago, when she began this brainstorming session, she told the assembled group of memory care residents, "Today we are coming up with big ideas. I'm going to share your thoughts with fourth graders at a nearby school. The students will use your ideas to create a play and later perform their work here at the care center."

She assured everyone that she welcomes all suggestions; there are no wrong answers.

Now Debra touches the sparkling gold top hat she wears, which is punctuated with a light bulb on its crown.

"Would you like to try my hat?" she asks Devin.

He opens one eye and nods. She places the hat on his head, and he looks absolutely kingly.

"New Year's Eve," he says, smiling.

"It does make you want to celebrate," Debra says. She shows him the vacuum tube. "Devin what else could we use this for?"

He puts it around his neck like a boa, and everyone laughs.

Bring Forth Big Ideas

Once a month, Debra visits this community and entices residents to explore their imaginations. She facilitates brainstorming sessions with a purpose: she wants to engage and energize the residents, and she also wants them to know she's going to use their ideas.

Today, she's lugged in a large cardboard box filled with props that she teases out one by one. A multicolored silky scarf is long enough to snake around the room so each of us can touch it.

"I had a jacket this color once," Marilyn tells me, stroking the royal blue silk.

> "As you think of new uses for familiar objects, you cheer each other on with positive feedback. The higher purpose is reminding your partners how much they have to give."

Debra brings out an umbrella and asks, "What could we do with this?"

"Twirl it," someone says.

"Hold it upside down and put something in it," another person offers.

Debra allows plenty of time for people to come up with ideas, and we applaud each person's creativity.

Although Debra often facilitates a group, her ideas work well with just two people. She usually has a theme for every session and tries to connect with each person through touch and by offering an object they can handle.

"You're engaging in the moment," Debra says. "As you think of new uses for familiar objects, you cheer each other on with positive feedback. The higher purpose is reminding your partners how much they have to give."

Creative Sparks

★ Put several easily recognizable items into a box or bag.

★ Tell your partner you want to think of new things to do with these familiar objects.

★ Explain that all ideas are welcome, the sillier the better.

★ Then ask your partner to pull out an object. If your partner doesn't recognize the object, you might say, "This is a spatula, normally used for cooking. What else could we use this for?" The open-ended questions invite creativity.

★ Allow plenty of time for contemplation. If needed, jump-start the creativity by offering your own thoughts.

★ Cheer on every idea.

★ Think of ways to use your brainstorming. For example, can you share them with family members and see how many suggestions they can add? Can you string them together and create a poem or a song? Can you make a guessing game out of your list, seeing if friends or family can guess what the object is?

CHAPTER NINE

Invite Creativity with Writing, Storytelling, and Poetry

Discover Your Own Personalized Poetic License

Prompt Imagination

Create Stories Together

Sneak Past the Facts and Connect through Poetry

Turn Ordinary Life into Extraordinary Poems

Honor Personal History

Celebrate Heroes through Storytelling and Scrapbooking

Discover Your Own Personalized Poetic License

"Storytelling is the most powerful way to put ideas into the world today." —Robert McKee

Mom read Shakespeare, and Dad recited Ogden Nash; that was the poetic division in our growing up household. Mom made up stories of talking schools of fish, and Dad regaled us with tales of shimmying up coconut trees in Panama. Toward the end of her life, Mom still remembered the challenges of being an Army nurse in Iceland and England during World War II, riding across the treacherous seas in a troop ship, working in a barracks-style hospital, and skiing to hot springs after hours. These scraps of adventure were her final stories.

During mom's journey through dementia, I often wrote down her words, realizing they might diminish, feeling they could be important to me later. I am so glad I have these mementos and have often shared them with family, friends, and others. In this chapter, writers and poets offer easy and comforting ways to invite out stories and creativity, through creating a safe place of acceptance and celebration.

Prompt Imagination

"Imagination is the highest kite that
one can fly." —Lauren Bacall

"Someone important has lost something valuable," Johnna Lowther from Kansas City, Missouri, tells her creative writing group. "Who is that someone?"

She stands poised to write as her group ponders this prompt.

"The person lives in Africa," one writer says.

"A lion," another adds.

"A lion queen, that's important," says someone else.

Johnna writes down each idea and then asks, "What did she lose?"

"Her supper."

"Her courage."

"Her cub."

"Yes, her cub." They all agree; the cub is lost. They murmur sympathetically.

"Where is he?" Johnna asks.

"A black snake captured him."

> "I learned early on that music, art, reading poetry, and writing really allow people with dementia to speak from the heart."

At the end of the writing session, everyone is buzzing with energy and laughter. Guided by Johnna's simple prompts, these eight people, who are living with dementia, smile as Johnna reads back their tall tale. Staff clusters closer, wanting to hear.

Johnna, who works as Director of Life Enrichment for Tutera Senior Living & Health Care, then reads the story back to the group, helping them once again celebrate the group synergy.

"I learned early on that music, art, reading poetry, and writing really allow people with dementia to speak from the heart," Johnna says. "Our goal is to write a story that each person contributes to. I simply jump-start the process by helping people lower their guard and get into a creative mode."

Creative Sparks

★ Come up with an evocative prompt, such as, "A man holds a key to something important. What is that important something? Who is the man?"

★ Invite imagination and welcome all ideas.

★ Acknowledge and write down each answer.

★ Ask additional questions, such as "Who will try to steal the key?" Periodically read aloud the answers so people can get a sense of the story.

★ Use this easy storytelling activity during meal times, car rides, visits, or family gatherings. You don't even need to write everything down; you can just enjoy the energy.

Create Stories Together

"The arts are so much more than a program—
they are a way of being in relationship, a way
of being in the world." —Anne Basting

Once Anne Basting encouraged imagination instead of memory, the stories started flowing. That fall of 1995, she was living in Milwaukee with a brand new PhD in theater studies. Every week, she volunteered in a nursing home, meticulously preparing dramatic exercises that invited people of varying mental and physical abilities to share specific memories. But the residents seemed too drugged, dazed, and confused to "talk about the sights, sounds, and aromas of Christmas."

After two months struggling to engage them, Anne decided to try something new. She cut out a picture of the Marlboro man from a magazine and showed the group the rugged-looking cowboy who was lighting up a cigarette.

"Forget about remembering," she said. "Let's make it up. What should we call this guy? Say anything, and I'll write it down."

"Fred," someone said.

Anne wrote it down.

"Fred who?" Anne asked.

"Fred Astaire," someone else answered. Several people laughed.

For forty-five minutes, Anne asked questions about Fred and his friends, and the residents answered, their imaginations soaring. Staff members wandered by, drawn in by the excited talking and laughing. At the end of the session, Anne had captured a far-reaching story that took place in Oklahoma and featured Fred and his wife Gina Autry, their three dogs, their black and white cows, and their rodeo-riding antics. She read the story to the group and everyone applauded.

The next week, Anne brought another picture and again asked open-ended questions. Another story emerged.

"Some of the words were nonsensical, but I took every comment seriously, writing it down and echoing it back. As I honored whatever the residents said, people became more comfortable talking. These creative conversations seemed to enhance their ability to communicate," Anne says.

Make Time to Imagine

"TimeSlips replaces the pressure to remember
with the invitation to imagine."

Building on these early sessions, Anne developed TimeSlips™ Creative Storytelling, which has become an award-winning, internationally acclaimed program. Family and professional care partners from around the world use TimeSlips™ concepts, and the nonprofit organization has now trained thousands of facilitators.

"TimeSlips replaces the pressure to remember with the invitation to imagine," Anne says. "This simple shift can balance the relationship between the care partners and the person living with dementia. By doing something creative and new together, you're focusing on strengths and participating as equals."

When your partner struggles to find the right words or stumbles over a phrase, many care partners feel an impulse to correct them, fill in the facts, and offer the answer. When that happens, your partner may revert to silence, worried her language is garbled or she's going to blurt out the wrong thing.

With TimeSlips™, people who have difficulty communicating can have fun with sounds, gestures, word fragments, and whole sentences.

"By doing something creative and new
together, you're focusing on strengths
and participating as equals."

Celebrate Self-Expression

The TimeSlips™ process does not depend on rational language or accurate memory. The experience works especially well with those who are beyond the early stages of dementia. Their creativity is frequently wide open.

"Radical listening" plays a large role in encouraging participants and developing the TimeSlips™ story. As she listens, Anne tries to mirror an individual's sounds, emotional intent, movements, and facial expressions.

One participant, Marge, only said, "bababa," in the sessions. Anne validated Marge's contribution by echoing the number of "bas," Marge's emotional tone, and her facial expressions. Within in weeks, Marge was inserting words between her "bababas," saying, "Bababa I love you bababa …"

"TimeSlips™ is open to all forms of expressions," Anne says. "All offerings are included in the story."

Sometimes they bring the story to life by working with a theater company, dance troupe, or other artistic team. That collaboration enriches the work, which may take the form of a dramatic reading, play, or movement piece.

Take TimeSlips™ Home

When Dr. Charles Farrell of Cleveland, Ohio, heard about TimeSlips™ on National Public Radio, he wanted to learn more. Luckily there was a training workshop for family care partners the next weekend. As Charlie sat in the workshop, learning how to use open-ended questions to invite out imagination instead of correcting memory, he had an "aha moment."

"I realized I'd been driving my wife crazy for the last two years," he said.

"I had to identify her ability, not her disability."

When his beloved wife Carol was diagnosed with dementia, Charlie's first impulse was to use his considerable medical skills, honed from forty years as a vascular surgeon, to try to cure her. But as he understood more about the TimeSlips™ process, he realized he needed to stop trying to fix Carol and focus on her strengths.

"That meant I had to identify her ability, not her disability," Charlie says. "I went from being a doctor who cured people to being someone who cared for people."

Use Stories to Stay Connected

Charlie was determined to keep Carol at home, connected with her family and community. TimeSlips™ helped him do that.

"We integrated the concepts at home, often using snapshots from family albums as the catalyst for our conversations," Charlie says.

Open-ended questions were key. Carol enjoyed socializing and looking at family pictures as long as she wasn't intimidated by having to remember names. Instead of asking, "Who's in this photo?" Charlie and the family members asked, "What does this look like to you?" Everyone participated in answering the questions. Sometimes they wrote down all the responses and created their own story; other times they just relished the creative unfolding.

"Looking at photos and inviting the imagination put visitors at ease and kept Carol engaged," Charlie says. "Those connections gave her life meaning and kept her involved with people."

Charlie also used TimeSlips™ in everyday conversations with Carol. They often walked around their neighborhood. One day Charlie said, "Tony's garden looks great this year."

Carol's face stiffened, and Charlie realized she didn't know who Tony was. He reframed his comment, reverting to an open-ended question. He pointed to Tony's home and said, "What do you think of that house?"

Carol smiled and said, "The house looks pretty, and those yellow flowers are fine, and I like seeing that black dog."

Help Others

"The key is learning how to communicate so each person feels honored and empowered."

Charlie treasures his ten years of caring for his wife.

"I got as much from Carol as she got from me," he says. "The key is learning how to communicate so each person feels honored and empowered."

TimeSlips™ inventor Anne Basting agrees.

"Using creativity tools, such as TimeSlips™, invites playful talk and laughter, and reduces tension and conflict," Anne says. "You also end up with a story you can share with others." Inspired by stories like Charlie's, TimesSlips™ now offers a creativity journal designed for family members to use at home.

Creative Sparks

★ Find visual images that offer an interesting juxtaposition of two things that don't belong together, such as a polar bear eating an ice cream cone or a small boy riding a penguin. Avoid photos that are too busy. You can also choose an interesting object, such as an old clock or vintage purse that may inspire ideas.

★ Engender a feeling of inclusion and openness by saying, "Let's make up a story about this image."

★ Use open-ended questions that invite imagination, such as "Where do you think they're going?" "How did they meet each other?" This gives people the freedom to participate without worrying about making mistakes.

★ Allow silence as needed. Give everyone plenty of time to respond.

★ Create TimeSlips™ stories one-on-one or invite others to join you. Take the process with you when you visit family or friends living with dementia. Use it during video communications, such as Skype or Zoom.

★ You can enjoy the experience without writing down the tale or you can capture it on paper or video and share it with others.

★ Visit the TimeSlips™ website (www.timeslips.org) for free software; there are more than 100 visual and question prompts. You can also invite family and friends to create a story with you by clicking on their "collaborate" button.

Sneak Past the Facts and Connect through Poetry

"Even in the late stages of dementia people can remember words and lines from poems they learned as children. Imagine how powerful it must feel to remember those words." —Gary Glazner

"Once upon a midnight dreary," Gary Glazner says, his voice rhythmic and melodic.

"Once upon a midnight dreary," we all repeat.

"While I pondered weak and weary," Gary says.

"While I pondered weak and weary," we echo.

I am attending Gary's Alzheimer's Poetry Project workshop in Santa Fe, New Mexico, and he is showing us how he uses the rhythm of poetry to engage with those living with memory loss. Gary, the author of *Dementia Arts*, travels the world, leading workshops through his nonprofit organization, The Alzheimer's Poetry Project.

"There are four steps to the process," Gary explains. "First, a call and response, where I read a line of verse and the group echoes it. After a stanza or two, we discuss the poem. Next, we add props to the experience, and finally we create our own poem."

Our group is a mixture of professional and family care partners and people living with dementia.

As Gary continues the second line of Poe's "The Raven," he notices a lady in a wheelchair who isn't participating. He walks up to her, kneels, and asks, "What is your name?"

"Betty," she says.

"May I take your hand?"

She nods.

"I'm going to recite a verse and I'll move your hand to the rhythm of the poem," he says.

He gently moves her hand from side to side as he recites, "Over many a quaint and curious volume of forgotten lore."

She smiles.

He stands and finishes the first stanza with call and response.

"Who has seen a raven?"

Several people raise their hand.

"What are ravens like?

"Big. Black. Bold." People throw out various answers.

Gary holds up two large ebony feathers.

"These are raven feathers," he says and passes them around the circle. The feather is stiff to the touch.

"Now we're going to create our own poem," Gary says. His assistant has a large, white tablet and is poised to write down every word.

"If you could fly, where would you go?"

The assistant writes down the answers: Paris, Kentucky, Antarctica, home, to see my children.

Betty says, "I would fly away from here."

"What does flying feel like?" Gary asks.

"Freedom. Angels. Clouds," people say.

When we've all spoken, Gary reads back our words. There's a sense of peace and grace in the room.

Gary's usual sessions last an hour. He centers his poems on a theme, such as summer, birds, trees, or food, and enriches the gathering with objects that engage the senses. For example, to supplement summertime creations, he might include a bucket of sand and a conch shell. He brings a misting spray to simulate an ocean breeze and lets people smell suntan lotion. For refreshments, he suggests fresh strawberries, lemonade, popsicles, or homemade ice cream.

"Poetry goes beyond the autobiographical memory and offers care partners a way to communicate with someone who has memory loss."

A study in the *American Journal of Physiology* documented the synchronization of heart rate and respiration during poetry recitation, showing the aerobic benefits of using the call and response technique in reciting poetry.

"Poetry goes beyond the autobiographical memory and offers care partners a way to communicate with someone who has memory loss," Gary says.

Creative Sparks

★ If your partner enjoys reading, print out familiar poems so you can then read them together.

★ Move your partner's hand to the rhythm of the recitation. This can be quite powerful, even in the late stages of dementia.

★ Include tactile and sensory accessories to bring the poems to life. You can add in aromas, fabric, music, and/ or a related food or drink.

★ Tailor the poems to your partner. For people in early stage, Gary recommends poems that can inspire conversations about their life. People in middle and later stages often engage with poems from their childhood.

★ Invite family and friends to a "poetry party." Choose a theme and invite people to bring copies of a favorite familiar poem to share. Connect with an icebreaker. Gary often incorporates a theater improv game called "Pass the smile." One person looks at another, smiles, and that person turns to the next, so the smile is silently passed around the circle. Take turns reading the poems, using the call and response.

★ A few of the familiar poems Gary uses include "The Tyger" by William Blake; "The Owl and the Pussy Cat" by Edward Lear; "Wynken, Blynken, and Nod" by Eugene Field; "How Do I Love Thee?" by Elizabeth Barrett Browning; "Purple Cow" by Gelett Burgess; "Jabberwocky" by Lewis Carroll; and "Daffodils" by William Wordsworth.

Turn Ordinary Life into Extraordinary Poems

"Value what people with dementia are saying, write it down, tape record it, affirm them when they say interesting or beautiful things because that's their personality showing through in a new way." —John Killick

John Killick identifies with Michelangelo's quote: "Every block of stone has a statue inside it and it is the task of the sculptor to discover it. I saw the angel in the marble and carved until I set him free."

Being engaged in writing a poem offers people self-expression, a feeling of purpose, the opportunity to learn new things, and a sense of achievement and well-being.

"My poetry creation process is like that," says John, who coauthored *Communication and the Care of People with Dementia* with Kate Allan. "When I work with people living with dementia, I amass a wad of words. I look at the central core and I edit away until the poem emerges."

Being engaged in writing a poem offers people self-expression, a feeling of purpose, the opportunity to learn new things, and a sense of achievement and well-being.

You're a Poet and Just Don't Know It

You don't need to be a poet or a big fan of poetry to facilitate or participate. John has developed a simple process that puts people at ease.

First, he reads aloud two classic works and one verse that is less familiar.

"I hand out copies of one, so people can notice how it's shaped on the page," John says. "Seeing the arrangement of words is part of understanding what a poem is."

After reading and discussing the writing, he says, "Let's make a poem."

> Asking open-ended questions is key to inviting out imagination.

The verse, he explains, isn't dictated by rhyme or meter; it's fueled by imagination and self-expression. He's learned that offering the group a subject, such as dogs, summer, or love doesn't work—the ideas generated are too scattered. Instead, he gives everyone a tangible stimulus to hold: old-timey sweets, a stone, or a photograph or painting with a simple, strong image. John stands ready with pen and paper, inviting people to comment on their objects.

"What do you feel about your picture or object?" he might ask. All answers are welcomed. Asking open-ended questions is key to inviting out imagination.

"Silly," says a woman who holds a picture of a goldfish. "Bubbly."

John writes down all words. He's relaxed and unhurried, giving people plenty of time to respond.

"What does your object remind you of?" John prompts.

Soon everyone is throwing out ideas, and John has a long list of phrases, words, and syllables. He reads the list aloud and says,

"This is our poem, but we haven't shaped it. We need a title, a first line, and a last line. What would be a good title?"

As a group, they decide which words and phrases to include and which to edit out. Once the writing is complete, he types it up and puts all the poets' names on the bottom. When the group meets again, John reads aloud their creation and hands everyone a copy. They then start the process again.

Finding the Angel, One-on-One

Sometimes people have an initial resistance to the idea of poetry. That happens when John works with a gentleman who lives in a dementia care community.

"I hate poetry," Ian initially informs John.

> "I wait for people to start talking. They will often come up with something unusual or close to their deepest concerns."

"Then we'll just have a conversation," John assures him.

John discusses what they'll be doing together. They're not focusing on remembering; they're creating something new. He'll be writing down the conversation but not engaging or interrupting; that way, the ideas can flow.

When meeting with an individual, John rarely uses any stimulus. "I wait for people to start talking," John says. "They will often come up with something unusual or close to their deepest concerns."

> "Creativity is essential to people with dementia. It bypasses the exercise of the intellect, provides valuable experiences, and enhances their sense of personhood."

John records his talk with Ian. Later, he hones in on its essence, editing out the extraneous words. He returns to Ian with a prose poem.

"My God," Ian says. "I'm a poet!"

John believes all people are poets. We just need someone to listen to them with curiosity and wonder, write down their words, and focus on what they're trying to express.

"A person with dementia may talk in a stream of conscious, meandering all over," John says. "It's not the transcriber's job to say, 'You're off the point,' because every tangent could be interesting."

Even though he's been orchestrating workshops for years, John is still amazed at the strength of the imaginative spirit and the quality of the poetry.

"Creativity is essential to people with dementia," John believes. "It bypasses the exercise of the intellect, provides valuable experiences, and enhances their sense of personhood."

Creative Sparks

★ Sit together in a quiet setting and discuss what you're doing to do. Tell your partner, "We're not focusing on remembering: we're creating something new. I'm going to write down what you say. I'm not going to reply or interrupt, so your words can really flow."

★ Then wait for your partner to talk. Let go of expectations and enjoy the unfolding.

★ Write or record every word. When there's a lull, read back the writing and ask if he'd like to say more.

★ Once the conversation is over, discover the focus by searching out repeated phrases and grouping similar thoughts.

★ Strengthen the impact of the piece by subtracting words and phrases that don't illustrate the theme. But don't add words. That way, the writing really belongs to the poet.

★ Type up the work and read it to the poet.

★ Celebrate by accumulating the writings and making a small book or sending friends "poem note cards."

Honor Personal History

"In the future everyone will be world-famous for fifteen minutes." —Andy Warhol

Imagine the frustration and anxiety of standing in the middle of the room, not knowing exactly where you are or who you are. A woman approaches you, walking slowly, smiling. She places a gentle hand on your arm and says, "You have been such a loving mother to your three daughters." You take a deep breath, feeling grounded and affirmed. You have been a loving mother. You have three daughters. Even if those facts do not stay in your mind, you have a moment of connection and recognition.

"When people can't tell their own stories, care partners can tell the stories for them."

"When people can't tell their own stories, care partners can tell the stories for them," says Tryn Rose Seley, author of *Fifteen Minutes of Fame.* She believes that offering such appreciations lifts the mood and boosts the energy of those living with dementia and their care partners. She has created a simple recipe for honoring lives, interests, and accomplishments, using stories, photos, affirmations, and songs to create a loving daily dose of "fifteen minutes of fame."

Search Out Stories

Her work with the elderly began in Pennsylvania as a home companion. When she moved to Colorado in 2002, she continued home health work, taking care of Ann, a woman who was living with dementia.

"I wanted to know more about Ann," Tryn says. "I noted information about her life through listening to her daughter's stories, noticing the photos Ann cherished, and paying attention to Ann's favorite songs. Then I brought those moments back to her."

Ann enjoyed being reminded of her life and accomplishments. When Tyrn retold Ann's significant stories, Ann's anxiety decreased, and she became happier and more communicative. So Tryn tried her idea with other clients and the results were equally rewarding.

Pick the Pictures

As she works with people living with memory loss, Tryn selects one or two photos that people view with affection, pictures that evoke a story. Then she says, "Tell me about this picture."

Sometimes, a significant picture is a catalyst.

She shows Fern a photo of a woman holding a baby and a hoe. "I have a story I'd like to tell you about when you were a young mother," she tells Fern, who sits up straight in her wheelchair and leans forward to look more closely at the black and white photo. "One day when your husband was at work and your daughter Emily was only a baby, you saw a black snake slither behind your kitchen stove . . ."

Fern grins. "I grabbed the baby and I got a hoe."

"You did. That was really quick thinking, by the way. Then . . ." Tryn waits to see if Fern wants to say more, but Fern is silent.

"Then," Tryn continues, "you marched back into that house . . ." Tryn finishes the tale of Fern bravely banishing the snake, and Fern says, "Then I sighed in relief and made us both a lemonade! Boy, that was some snake."

Write Out Affirmations

Tryn also supports her clients by creating affirmation cards, stating a significant life event, such as "You have made women beautiful by your clothing designs. Thank you," or "You became a judge and made a difference in people's lives. Thank you." She places the card at the breakfast table or on the bathroom mirror. Tryn speaks of these happy memories throughout the day, building feelings of connection and trust.

Know That Tune

Tryn writes down the lyrics to clients' favorite songs. Then, if they are depressed, disoriented, or stuck in a repetitive loop, Tryn hands over the lyrics and starts singing the familiar tune. Often, they'll sing along.

For those who play musical instruments, Tryn recommends keeping a list of their favorite tunes nearby. That way, someone can request a song, igniting the powerful connection between memory and music.

Creative Sparks

★ Listen to the stories your partner tells. Consider the accomplishments she prizes and the relationships she cherishes.

★ Ask friends and family for their favorite stories about your partner. Test those stories out and see if there's a positive response.

★ Set the stage by saying, "I have a story I'd like to tell you about a time when you were living on the farm," or "Can I tell you about the time when . . . ?" Keep the stories brief and focused on your partner.

★ Laminate two or three photos that illustrate important moments in your partner's life. Use these to anchor your partner's sense of self and to start conversations.

★ Support significant events with affirmation cards, stating the achievement and thanking them. You can simply print on an index card, "You were a beloved kindergarten teacher and you helped so many children. Thank you."

★ Place these cards in prominent locations, so you can notice and talk about them during the day.

Celebrate Heroes through Storytelling and Scrapbooking

"Each of us has a family tree full of stories inside
of us . . . Each of us has a story blossoming
out of us." —Francesca Lia Block

What could I do to keep my mom engaged and creative? I wondered. She snubbed her usual passions of drawing, gardening, or swimming. She couldn't concentrate enough to read. She was too restless to sit through a movie.

While I was trying to come up with an activity, I was missing my daughter Sarah who had recently moved away to college. I decided to make a story-scrapbook for Sarah starring the giant red plush Elmo she'd left behind. I invited Mom to be part of *Some Things You Don't Know about Elmo.*

Celebrating and Engaging Everyday Heroes

Thus, the HERO Project was born, a simple story brought to life in a scrapbook-style notebook, celebrating someone living with dementia. This easy and engaging artistic endeavor enhances self-esteem, creativity, and interaction.

I wrote a quick story about the secret life of Elmo. Mom and I discussed photo opportunities, and her standard, "Whatever," sounded more upbeat then usual. We laughed a lot during the photo shoot, Mom giggling as she dressed Elmo in one of Sarah's old party dresses and a purple wig. Then she propped him in a chair and held open his *Wall Street Journal*. She settled Elmo in the refrigerator so he could sneak a snack and chuckled as she sat in the passenger seat with Elmo behind the wheel.

After the photos were developed, Mom helped me choose the best ones. Then we pasted them with accompanying storylines into a scrapbook. Mom searched through magazines for jaunty pictures to liven up the pages. For several hours, I reveled in the enjoyable feeling of working on a creative mission with my mom.

Thus, the HERO Project was born, a simple story brought to life in a scrapbook-style notebook, celebrating someone living with dementia. This easy and engaging artistic endeavor enhances self-esteem, creativity, and interaction.

Using HERO Projects to Connect

When Ron's father, Frank, moved to a care home, we wanted to honor Frank with a HERO book. We chose the theme of *Lucky Frank* and wrote a short personal history, an homage to Frank's long and serendipitous life. We mentioned family, friends, quirks, accomplishments, and dementia in the story and photos.

When Frank moved from assisted living into memory care, we used his HERO book, *Lucky Frank,* so his new care team could get to know him as a person.

"Even though Frank could no longer remember all his adventures," we wrote, "he is still lucky enough to continue to have adventures." With Frank's permission, we shared the finished product with the staff and family.

When Frank moved from assisted living into memory care, we used his HERO book, *Lucky Frank*, so his new care team could get to know him as a person. The book stayed in his room, and we often used it to jump-start a visit. Frank always enjoyed reading or looking at his story. This simple book gave us all, particularly Frank, a lot of pleasure.

Creative Sparks

★ Come up with a theme and a storyline based on your partner's personal history, milestones, or hobbies.

★ Write a simple script. This is not about literary excellence; you're trying to capture a small part of the person's life.

★ Share the storyline with your partner and ask for feedback.

★ Consider how you will illustrate your story and orchestrate a photo shoot. Choose a well-lit setting at a time that works for your partner, energy-wise. Bring props, music, and snacks to make the experience exhilarating.

★ Print or develop the best photos and print the story.

★ Have a little collage party and scrapbook the pages.

★ Give people living with dementia as much power as possible over their pages. People who can't speak or aren't able to handle the materials can still be involved. Just show them a picture and give them choices of where you might put the photo on the page.

★ Share the completed story by reading it aloud and displaying the finished product. Make copies as needed.

CHAPTER TEN

Express Yourself through the Arts

It's Almost like Being in Love

Open Your Imagination by Looking at Art

Visit a Gallery and Draw on Memory

Brush Away Apathy through Painting

Draw One Line, Then Another

Bring Imagination into the Picture

Open Studios Invite Artistic Exploration

Illustrate Your Life

Weave In Fabric

Connect through Collage

Cut, Paste, and Converse

It's Almost like Being in Love

"Art washes away from the soul the dust
of everyday life." —Pablo Picasso

I remember the first time I saw Van Gogh's painting *Starry Night*. My mother had checked out a book of Impressionist art from the Memphis Public Library, and we poured over it together. My breath caught when I saw the midnight blue swirls, and I was swept into the vortex of color and imagination. Van Gogh's *Bedroom at Arles* and *Sunflowers* lifted my spirits and ignited my dreams.

> "Because people living with dementia express what they think and feel at the moment, they are natural artists and natural audiences for artistic expression."

John Zeisel, PhD, understands the transformative effect of viewing art. Working through his *I'm Still Here Foundation*, which serves those living with dementia, John and his colleague Sean Caulfield, MEd, founded *Artists for Alzheimer's* or *ARTZ* in 2002, which, ten years later, grew into the community transformation program *It Takes a Village*. They approached MoMA, where they designed a tour especially for people living with dementia and their care partners. They created an art-viewing program in Europe, starting with tours at the Louvre. They also developed a template so they could share this program with other galleries. Today museums all over the world emulate these tours.

"Because people living with dementia express what they think and feel at the moment, they are natural artists and natural audiences for artistic expression," John says. "Art touches and engages the brain in profound ways. People living with dementia endure a lot of loss, and the arts can provide meaningful connections to their emotions, their culture, and their communities."

Looking at visual art is not just a passive activity; it's an act of creative observation and a catalyst for conversation and learning. Plus, seeing magnificent works of art makes us happy. According to research by Semir Zeki, Professor of Neuroesthetics at University College London, experiencing a beautiful work of art and feeling love both create the feel-good chemical dopamine in our brains.

Art Matters

Frank sits in his wheelchair, arms folded across his chest, gazing quietly into the distance. He doesn't seem to register the other people seated around the long table. He doesn't appear to notice the container of watercolors and the bowl of water to his left. But when the facilitator puts a paintbrush into his

> "The act of painting can unlock memories, stimulate thoughts, and promote social interaction."

hand and says, "Want to paint something, Frank?" he instantly dips the brush into the water, swabs the blue paint, and begins. He paints a bright face that looks like businessman-turned-clown and a mountain that glows like a southwest sunset. He doesn't know the date or time or that he once studied architecture. He doesn't always remember how many sons he has or where he lives. But he can paint with a verve and freedom that he couldn't access when he was younger.

"Even after memory and cognitive functions are damaged, the ability to create art can continue," says Karen Clond, LMSW, Heart of America Alzheimer's Association in Prairie Village, Kansas. "Creativity springs from the areas of the brain that process emotion, and we know that emotions such as fear, love, attachment, and appreciation of beauty continue to live in the person with Alzheimer's disease. These feelings sometimes find their expression in art. The act of painting can unlock memories, stimulate thoughts, and promote social interaction."

The Alzheimer's Association began its Memories in the Making art project in 1988, and now chapters across the country offer the program. Facilitators create a safe and encouraging atmosphere so the participants can explore painting with watercolors as a failure-free activity.

You don't need special artistic abilities to facilitate and enjoy the ideas in this chapter. Plus, there's a bonus in integrating art into your lives: While you're painting, you may also be brushing away dementia. A 2015 Mayo Clinic study found participants who engaged in artistic hobbies such as painting, drawing, or sculpture in both middle and old age were 73 percent less likely to develop mild cognitive impairment than those who didn't. Viewing and creating art are ways to increase happiness, conversation, cognition, and connection.

Open Your Imagination by Looking at Art

"Art has the power to transform, to illuminate, to educate, inspire, and motivate." —Harvey Fierstein

For Gloria, the brief journey from her mother's bedroom to the memory unit's community area seems endless.

"Where are we going?" her mother, Irene, asks. "I don't want to go. I am so confused. Where are we going? I don't want to go."

"We're going to look at art, Mom," Gloria says. "It'll be fun."

When Gloria finally settles her mom into a chair, Irene cocoons into herself and seems oblivious of the other people in the circle. Even though Irene formerly loved going to galleries and museums, she doesn't stir when the facilitator asks, "How many of you enjoy looking at art?"

The facilitator strolls over to Irene, gently gets her attention, and shows her a Norman Rockwell print featuring a young girl and a dog.

Irene stares at the picture.

"What do you see?" asks the facilitator.

"I had a dog," Irene says. "Peaches."

"Tell us about Peaches."

"She loved to catch balls," Irene says. "She slept with me."

"I had a dog named Happy," says another woman.

"My brother had a spaniel," says a man.

"Peaches was a terrier," Irene says.

Gloria takes a deep breath and smiles as her mother chats about her dog and interacts with the others. The art invited Irene out, and Irene's conversation connected her with others.

"Looking at art and making observations gives people living with dementia a chance to exercise their imagination and creativity," says Susan Shifrin, PhD, Director, ARTZ Philadelphia. "Many people with dementia have a heightened sensitivity and openness to art, even if they had no previous artistic aptitude."

> "Looking at art and making observations gives people living with dementia a chance to exercise their imagination and creativity."

Prior to a museum visit, an ARTZ facilitator may bring photos of familiar masterpieces to a care community, noticing which pictures evoke memories, emotions, and conversation. The facilitator then tailors the tour to feature similar pieces. Even galleries without a special ARTZ program may design visits for those who are living with dementia.

Art Invites Conversation

> "Going to cultural activities offers people a sense of normalcy and gives them a date to put on their calendars."

Teri Miller, with the Alzheimer's Association-Houston & Southeast Texas Chapter, has witnessed the power of creativity and the arts. As the Early-Stage Program Manager, Teri collaborates with a variety of Houston's arts and civic organizations.

"Going to cultural activities offers people a sense of normalcy and gives them a date to put on their calendars," she says. "When they go with friends or care partners, they have an experience to discuss. Even people who say, 'Oh, I don't care for museums,' usually have a great time."

Sam is an example of someone who was surprised to enjoy the art gallery.

He attended one of Teri's early stage support groups. His wife, who cared for him at home, went to the care partner's group. Teri formed a partnership with the Houston Museum of Fine Arts and invited her early stage group to experience a tour with their care partners. When he heard the invitation, Sam rolled his eyes and said, "I've never been to a museum and I'm not about to start now."

But the next week, Sam signed up for the tour.

"What made you change your mind?" Teri asked.

"My wife really wanted to go. She does so much for me, I figured I'd do something for her."

Teri expected Sam to sit back silently, arms folded over his chest, then the docent asked, "What does this painting make you think of? Has anyone ever been in a similar setting?" But to Teri's surprise, Sam had opinions on each of the three pieces they discussed.

Sam's wife smiled as Sam told Teri, "At first, I didn't want to go because I was worried I wouldn't have anything meaningful to contribute. But I guess you don't have to know anything about art to enjoy the museum."

He and his wife talked about the experience all the way home. Discussing the paintings opened up chances to reminisce and connect. Plus, the experience gave them something interesting to share with their grown children and visiting neighbors.

Like many art partnerships around the country, Teri was inspired by MoMA's Meet Me art program for people living with dementia. The Houston museum benefitted from MoMA coming to train their docents. The program offers comprehensive guidelines for visiting a museum or viewing art at home.

Creative Sparks

Many art galleries and museums offer special tours and events for people living with dementia. If you're lucky enough to have such a tour available, take advantage of it.

To design your own museum tour:

★ Think of a museum your partner likes. If feasible, buy postcards of some of its art or visit its online gallery together and ask your partner which pieces he prefers. That way, you can tailor the visit to his taste.

★ Choose one or two rooms that feature his preferred art. Make sure one room has a place to sit.

★ Use the paintings and sculptures as a catalyst for conversation. Ask open-ended questions, discussing the colors, people, and objects you both notice.

★ If the museum has a restaurant or tearoom, treat yourselves to something delicious.

★ Enjoy the sense of connection that comes from discussing art; there are no right or wrong answers, just interesting observations.

To fashion a viewing experience at home:

★ Select art books from the library or use your own personal collection.

★ Choose works that portray emotion, tell a story, or align with your partner's background or interests.

★ Ask open-ended questions that invite conversation, such as, "What does this make you think of?" and "What do you notice in this picture?" Have fun imagining what the people in the painting are thinking. Imagine their professions and whether they're happy.

Visit a Gallery and Draw on Memory

"Painting is by nature a luminous language." —Robert Delaunay

"I want us to explore this work of art together," Laura Voth says. As we settle in chairs facing the large painting, she passes out small copies of this Leon Kroll work titled *Lower New York, The Bridge in Winter, 1915*. Today's oil features an old-fashioned Manhattan skyline as seen from underneath a bridge. Several boats navigate a choppy river.

Laura is education assistant at the Philbrook Museum of Art in Tulsa, Oklahoma. Ron and I have joined today's Focus on Art program, a collaboration between the Philbrook and the Alzheimer's Association, Oklahoma Chapter. The experience is for people living with dementia and their care partners and is designed to help them connect with art using imagination and observational skills.

Laura offers our group of fifteen a little background on the painting and then asks, "What do you see in the painting?"

"Lots of big buildings," Thomas says.

"What can you tell me about those buildings?" Laura asks.

"Tall," Thomas says.

"It looks like New York, but I've never seen it from this angle," Julie says.

I realize I, too, have never seen New York from that angle and I start noticing a few more of the picture's details: two tug boats bouncing around in the rough waves and several men hoisting a rope from a dock.

"Has anyone been to New York?" Laura asks.

"We marched through there and got right on a boat," Thomas says.

"What would it be like on that boat?" Laura asks.

"I can't swim," Julie says.

"I've been to New York as a visitor," Mary says.

The conversation continues as Laura asks other observational questions about the picture, "What time of year do you think it is? Does the painting make you feel small or tall? What do you think that round building is? What would you put in that round building?"

Everyone participates, treating each question with curiosity.

After the conversation, we go downstairs to create our own art.

In the art room, each person has a large sheet of drawing paper, which is easy to see against the dark green table cover. The team from the Alzheimer's Association works with the museum staff, making sure each person is comfortable and can reach the supplies. Laura shows us how to draw simple lines and sketch a bridge and then guides us in drawing squares for houses, triangles for roofs, and circles for ponds.

At the end, Emily has a wonderfully vibrant painting to take home, and I have a wonderfully vibrant feeling from connecting with an interesting woman.

I'm sitting across from Emily, who looks blankly at the paintbrushes and says, "I can't draw."

I ask what color she likes.

"Orange," she says.

I show her the orange paint and ask if she'd like to try some.

She dips in her brush and strokes paint across the paper.

Color by color, she asks, "What now? What color shall I use? Where does this color go?"

During our painting session, I learn she was born in West Virginia, she doesn't like to cook, she has five children, and her brother is a wood carver. One of her treasured possessions is a statue of Dopey her brother carved when he was a teenager.

At the end, Emily has a wonderfully vibrant painting to take home, and I have a wonderfully vibrant feeling from connecting with an interesting woman.

Creative Sparks

★ You don't need to be an artist or have previous experience to enjoy painting projects.

★ Lay out the supplies. Crayons and watercolors work well. For a unique look, paint over a white crayon.

★ Sit by your partner and help her get started. If she hesitates, you may simply ask, "What color do you want to try, purple or orange?"

★ Encourage her to stay engaged. If she falters, ask a question about what color or shape she'd like to try next. While she works, make your own art.

Brush Away Apathy through Painting

"The power of art is transformative." —Berna Huebner

"I remember better when I paint," Berna Huebner's mother said to her one day. Despite that statement, Berna's mom, Hilgos, who had been a successful artist, was often detached, indifferent, and slumped into a morass of forgetfulness. Berna was in despair, not knowing how to revive her lively, talented mother. The staff at the memory care facility seemed to think her mom's behavior was just the normal course of the disease, but Berna felt differently. She was determined to unearth her mother from the puddle of apathy and engage her once again in the painting she loved.

"I remember better when I paint."

It took months of persistent encouragement before Berna's mother finally picked up a brush and began painting again. Berna engaged area art students in the project. Almost every day, a student set out watercolor supplies. The student painted a line and offered Hilgos the brush. Day after day, Hilgos simply ignored the student, who sat nearby, painting, chatting, and gently inviting Hilgos to participate. Then one day, Hilgos took the brush and painted a line. Another day, she kept the brush and painted a picture. Gradually, she returned to the art she so loved, creating bright and exciting pictures. More importantly, she replenished her self-esteem and interest in life.

To help others connect through art, Berna worked with Eric Ellena, codirecting a documentary, *I Remember Better When I*

Paint. She also edited a book with the same name. She founded the Hilgos Foundation, which helps people living with dementia reconnect with themselves through art.

"Doctors in the film and book say that parts of the brain are spared; therefore, people with memory impairment can express themselves through the creative arts," Berna says.

Creative Sparks

★ Try different types of art in different venues to see what resonates with your partner.

★ To add extra meaning, connect the artistic activity with something in your partner's past.

★ Invite an intergenerational mixture of artists, such as children, grandchildren, art students, and volunteers to join your partner and add encouragement.

★ Create a variety of art-related activities, including visiting galleries or looking at pictures from magazines, as well as painting, drawing, or various media.

★ Don't give up. The artistic process can take time.

Draw One Line, Then Another

"Dementia is not scary like most people think. I
find working with people with dementia to be
creative and really fun. Their hearts and souls
are always intact." —Shelley Klammer

"What color do I put here?" Margaret asks, her voice anxious. She looks uncertainly at artist and facilitator Shelley Klammer, who is next to her in the care home's dining room.

"Which color do you prefer?" Shelley asks.

Margaret wrings her hands and does not answer. She is living with dementia and has been recently rescued from a neglectful situation.

"Do you like green or purple?" Shelley asks, pointing to the two colors of paint.

Margaret nods toward the purple. Shelley dabs a brush in the purple watercolor and demonstrates how to paint within a pre-drawn outline of a flower. She hands the brush to Margaret, who copies her example.

"What color shall we use next?" Shelley asks.

"Research is now recognizing how making art
soothes and engages people with dementia.
Imagery often expresses what words cannot."

Margaret points to the red. Shelley continues painting with Margaret for several sessions, until Margaret begins picking out her own colors. For Margaret, this one-on-one invitation to make art evolves into a passion for painting within pre-drawn familiar patterns, such as animals, flowers, and trees. Margaret has grown calmer since she started painting, smiling the whole time she makes art.

"Research is now recognizing how making art soothes and engages people with dementia," Shelley says. "Imagery often expresses what words cannot. A pre-drawn structure allows an anxious painter to relax into the process. Painting familiar subject matter can help a person with dementia settle into a pleasurable, meditative state."

Art Brings Benefits

Many people shy away from art, disillusioned by negative grade school experiences, believing they can't draw. But artists with dementia often forget such early criticism.

"Creativity can increase with the onset of dementia."

"Creativity can increase with the onset of dementia," Shelley says. "It's as though the censorship button has been turned off. A painter with dementia often feels a freedom to choose unconventional colors like purple grass or a green sky."

Shelley is an artist, therapist, and the author of the e-book, *How to Start an Art Program for the Elderly*. For years, she worked in Canada's largest therapeutic art studio with adults who were living with late stage dementia or other physical and mental issues. Some of the benefits she's witnessed include increases in attention span, enhanced self-awareness and self-esteem, memory stimulation, and the calming of anxiety disorders.

Structure Invites Creativity

Shelley tries to make each art experience a treasured time.

"The frail elderly don't necessary feel the need to accomplish a sophisticated end product," Shelley says. "Many create for the sake of feeling connected. They may primarily seek the respect, acknowledgment, and encouragement that accompany the process."

A familiar setting and routine help ease people into art. Shelley uses classical and meditative music as a cue to relax and settle in. To get people interested, she often instigates an "artistic conversation," drawing a line and inviting her partner to add a line. Then she draws another. She uses good quality watercolors and weaves in topics of personal interest to the artist, such as flowers, cats, or farm scenes. Once a person begins painting on her own, Shelley lets her be, stifling any urge to instruct.

"Then it's time to appreciate. Describe what you like about your partner's picture," Shelley says. "For example, 'I like the way you streaked the green through the sky. I like the white space you left in the center.'"

Shelley shares her own piece of art and asks for comments then thanks her partner for joining her, offering extra affirmations as appropriate. For example, "Thanks for telling me about your rose garden. Thank you for sharing that interesting story about horses." Those affirmations complete the circle of connection until the next time.

Inspire Creativity by Making Gifts

Making projects they can give as presents to family and friends is a big motivation for many people living with dementia. For an ongoing project that will last for several art sessions, Shelley suggests buying a wooden box or birdhouse at a craft store. Using acrylics, Shelley guides her art partners in painting the structure with a single color, such as green. After the initial coat dries, they make vertical stripes with thick masking or painter's tape and repaint the entire object a different color, such as blue. When that dries, they peel off the tape and revel in the two-tones. Later, they add any other decorations, such as small colorful pebbles or pretty collage papers and then many coats of varnish.

Other artists might enjoy creating hand-painted watercolor papers or using ink stamps to decorate paper. They can then use the paper to make and write gift cards. Or they can cut up the colored papers into smaller shapes and collage the shapes onto blank cards. Painting on T-shirts, caps, and tote bags offer other options.

The Spontaneous Session

Shelley has spent thousands of hours working with elder artists. In the beginning, she over-prepared, but nothing ever turned out as she'd planned.

"I learned to go with the flow," Shelley says. "I engaged each person at his or her level and let go of my preset list of objectives. If they want to paint the masking tape around the picture and it gives them the pleasure of deeply concentrated attention, we go with that. I try not to over-direct."

As long as everyone in the art group feels seen, heard, and acknowledged in their unique personhood, Shelley deems the art session a success.

As long as everyone in the art group feels seen, heard, and acknowledged in their unique personhood, Shelley deems the art session a success.

Creative Sparks

★ Designate a "creative corner" for your art space. This can be as simple as the kitchen table.

★ Follow the same routine each time, such as turning on some relaxing music, sharing a cup of tea, and beginning a conversation about the art materials.

★ Provide a starting point by using geometric or familiar structures. Staring at a blank page can be intimidating for anyone.

★ Make a "mandala" by tracing around a saucer or plate, so there's a welcoming circle on the page.

★ Partner paint, taking turns making marks, until your partner is creating on her own. Then you can quietly pull back and work on your own art alongside.

★ Explore projects you can give to loved ones, such as painted boxes, birdhouses, picture frames, or cards.

★ Make the experience special. You might include a classic painting or popular poster to look at and discuss, along with a cup of tea and a delicious cookie.

★ Thank your partner for contributing and acknowledge his efforts. Appreciate yourself as well.

Bring Imagination into the Picture

"When words become unclear, I shall focus with photographs. When images become inadequate, I shall be content with silence." —Ansel Adams

"Photograph what you love and love what you photograph," the teacher said. She'd put together a short slide show, featuring photos of family, travel, food, and nature and invited conversation on each topic. Then she talked a little about light and texture and handed out disposable cameras.

"Have fun taking pictures," she told her students, who were part of Teri Miller's Early Onset Group through the Houston Alzheimer's Association.

The participants had concrete proof of their creativity.

Richard already had a list of photographs he wanted to take. He was especially interested in capturing photos of his grandfather's farm, where he'd spent many summers as a boy. The photography assignment gave Richard and his daughter a focus for the week. One day, his daughter drove him sixty miles to see the old house his grandfather used to own. It looked forlorn and abandoned out there, surrounded by fields, but it also brought up a lot of memories and feelings for Richard. He talked about his childhood with great passion, and his daughter heard several new stories. He was so moved by the visit that he wrote a poem to accompany the photos.

At the next meeting, the teacher collected the cameras. She had the pictures blown up and created an art show, as well as a booklet of each person's photos. The participants had concrete proof of their creativity; something to display, discuss, and share.

"They'd had a chance to express themselves and their faces shone with pleasure," Teri says.

Point and Shoot Together

> "The person living with dementia doesn't need to know how to use the camera; you can work together to create ideas and compositions and decide what photos to take."

Cameras can be a tool for exploration and experimentation. Claire Craig, author of *Exploring the Self through Photography*, uses pictures to spark imaginative enquiry. She might ask, "What do you notice? What do you think this place smells like? What are these people or animals doing?"

After talking about the pictures, Claire and the other photographers choose a theme for a photo shoot, such as favorite birds, preferred fruits, or garden flowers. Or they take a walk and see what inspires them. If it's too hard to venture outdoors, they bring bits of the garden in and set up still lifes.

"The person living with dementia doesn't need to know how to use the camera; you can work together to create ideas and compositions and decide what photos to take," Claire says. Claire likes to print out the results as soon as possible. She invites participants to help her sort through photos. She preserves the pictures in frames, photo albums, scrapbooks, greeting cards, and postcards.

Make the Ordinary into an Extraordinary Picture

A large crowd gathers for the opening of the Silverado Photo Project exhibit in Los Angeles, California. One of the featured photographers asks the event coordinator, "Are my sons here yet? Do you think they'll be proud of me?"

His sons are not just proud; they are amazed at the creativity and clarity of their father's photographs. When they were growing up, their dad always had a camera in hand. But since his dementia diagnosis, he hasn't taken any pictures. This photo project reconnects him with a life passion.

> "It was wonderful to see the residents' pride and self esteem as their work was displayed in a prestigious downtown gallery."

The concept of the project is simple and easy to replicate. At the five Los Angeles Silverado Memory Care communities, several professional photographers partnered with Canon and offered the residents the use of digital cameras.

They encouraged the budding photographers to take pictures inside and outside of their care communities. The professionals offered guidance as needed and frequently showed residents the pictures they've just snapped, so they received instant feedback. Some had never held a camera; others were known as the family photographer.

After five weeks, the professionals culled through the photos, framed some, and put together a show. The residents and staff invited friends, family, and the public.

Each photo was part of a silent auction, and they raised $6,000 for the Los Angeles chapter of the Alzheimer's Association.

"It was wonderful to see the residents' pride and self-esteem as their work was displayed in a prestigious downtown gallery," says Kathy Greene, Senior Vice President of Program and Services Integration, Silverado Memory Care. "Plus, showing their artistic abilities educates the community on how creative people living with dementia can be."

Keep Clicking

When taking pictures, photographer Cathy Greenblat offers this advice: "Keep clicking. It always takes many shots to capture a great picture. Plus, as people get used to seeing you using the camera, they feel more at ease."

Cathy Greenblat, PhD, had taken an early retirement from her career as a professor of sociology. She decided to deepen her knowledge of photography by taking a master class with a renowned documentary photographer in Oaxaca, Mexico. Her teacher's assignment did not please Cathy: go to the local old age home and take pictures.

> "I knew I had something powerful, a message
> about seeing dementia differently and
> understanding what people could accomplish
> in a supportive and creative environment."

Cathy had had too many negative experiences in care homes: both her grandparents had lived with dementia and had languished in long-term care. The last thing she needed was to revisit those bad memories. "I wanted to tell my instructor this assignment was all wrong for me," Cathy says.

Cathy overcame her resistance and visited the home. She talked to the people living there and captured their energy and essence through her photography. The instructor loved Cathy's work and urged her to continue photographing the elderly.

That summer, while she was staying in California, a friend offered to take Cathy to visit a dementia care community. Cathy reluctantly agreed. When she toured the community, she realized this company provided gold standard care, treating people with dignity and compassion; the residents were lively and engaged. Cathy received permission to photograph, and she spent the next seven weeks there, taking pictures, hanging out, interviewing, and listening. She got to know the residents and staff well, and she captured the interactions that made the community so special. At the end of her visit, she had thousands of pictures.

"My husband cried every time I showed him new images," she says. "I knew I had something powerful, a message about seeing dementia differently and understanding what people could accomplish in a supportive and creative environment." She used about ninety of the photos in her book *Alive with Alzheimer's* and the related exhibit that toured internationally.

Since 2004 she has traveled the world, taking uplifting photos of people living with dementia in eleven countries. The result is her internationally acclaimed book, *Love, Loss, and Laughter: Seeing Alzheimer's Differently*, filled with compelling text and 110 vibrant images. The parallel exhibit has been hosted at many galleries, including those at the United Nations, the World Health Organization Headquarters, and the National Academy of Sciences.

"Through my visits to private homes, day programs, and residential communities, I saw that many capacities remain despite the losses that come with dementia," Cathy says. "It's up to us to nurture those capacities. I hope my photos help others change their minds about people's changing brains and keep love and joy alive."

Creative Sparks

★ Learn as much as you can about your partner and her current interests. The more you know about the person living with dementia, the better you can guide her in her photography.

★ Show your partner how to use the camera and together choose a theme or a focus.

★ If the camera presents problems for your partner, discuss what photos to take. Then you click the camera.

★ Take more photos than you need. Good pictures are hard to take.

★ Set up a multigenerational photography project involving your partner, family members, and friends. Ask a knowledgeable friend to offer you simple photographic advice.

★ Use the photo-taking as a way to trigger and deepen conversations.

★ Share the photos as soon as possible with your partner.

★ Offer to print them out, mount a show in your home, or turn the photos into postcards.

Open Studios Invite Artistic Exploration

"Imagination embraces the entire world, and all there ever will be to know and understand." —Albert Einstein

When artist Jeff Nacthigall walks into the art studio for a session with people living with dementia, he feels he's working with his peers. He knows he's going to learn from them, and he hopes to help these emerging artists make their authentic mark. Jeff doesn't believe in teaching art. He doesn't use coloring books or crafts. He hands artists a blank page, knowing initially he may encounter some resistance.

Jeff has seen people with dementia emerge from a shell of indifference and isolation into a blaze of artistic expression.

"We are all born artists," Jeff says. "But our expressive spirit often is tamped down or ignored. When we communicate through the arts, we can become quite creative."

Jeff has seen people with dementia emerge from a shell of indifference and isolation into a blaze of artistic expression.

Jeff works within long-term care facilities and other communities and designs Open Studios, safe spaces to experiment with and produce art. The Open Studio Project began in his home country of Canada and has since spread throughout the world. Jeff's philosophy is "push aside limitations and concentrate on strengths." He spent years concentrating on his own strengths after he experienced a brain injury as a teenager. For him, the artistic process is about recognizing people's barriers and charting a course through them.

To help people move past resistance and embrace their artistic nature, Jeff suggests some of these warm ups.

Paint Pour

Jeff puts a small amount of acrylic paint into a cup and invites the artists to pour the paint over a cardboard box or wooden block. They observe the way the paint drips and puddles on the three-dimensional objects. They can also pour onto a canvas or piece of paper. They move the canvas or paper from side to side, holding it upright to encourage paint flow. Then they add other colors. Pouring is a recognized form of contemporary art and is a playful way to engage people and produce fascinating paintings.

Sponge and Roll

For another freeing way to spark art, Jeff's artists slip on plastic work gloves, dip tennis balls in paint, and roll them around on paper or canvas.

Squirt

Jeff fills a water pistol or squeeze bottle with watercolor or diluted acrylic and invites the artist to squirt it on the page. They then tilt the paper in various directions for artistic drips.

Combine Techniques

Layering invites an ongoing project. Artists sponge on one color and let it dry, then squirt on a new color. After drying, they roll on the next color.

"We're building creative capacity," Jeff says. "These mindful artistic activities can bring forth passion and joy."

Creative Sparks

★ Clear your mind of expectations. Think about playing and having fun.

★ Expect initial resistance and be open to trying and trying again.

★ Explore different ways to invite people to make their mark on a page. For inspiration, look at contemporary art.

★ Experiment with paint pouring, squirting, and sponging.

★ Be patient. People may be slow to make a simple mark on the blank page; it's important to give them time.

Illustrate Your Life

"A picture is a poem without words." —Horace

"I'm creating a mural, featuring important elements of people's lives," Australian artist Julie Gross McAdam, PhD, explains to Dorothy, an elder in the memory care unit. "What would you like me to include about you in the painting?"

"I had a little dog," Dorothy answers.

Dorothy describes her beloved pet, and Julie jots down notes.

Later, Julie drops by to visit Dorothy, bringing acrylic paints and a sketch that includes the small dog.

"I've outlined your dog," Julie says to Dorothy, pointing to the drawing. "What color was his coat?"

"Brown."

Julie hands Dorothy a paintbrush with brown paint on it. Dorothy holds the brush for a moment and then begins painting in the dog. Julie invites her to color in other portions of the drawing, which include a cottage, fence, and garden. When Dorothy's daughter arrives, she paints "Penny," the dog's name, on its collar.

"For some, picking up the brush, dipping it into paint, and stroking it across the paper is too many steps," Julie says. So I simplify the process by putting the paint on the brush."

For people who can't use the brush, Julie puts their hand on top of hers while she paints so they can feel the movement of the brush. Regardless of the artistic results, the act of sitting close to someone while painting is engaging.

Creativity Rules

"I've never met someone who is not creative, who could not enjoy some art form. We all take joy in making things look beautiful," Julie says. In addition to being an artist, Julie is also a respected gerontologist. She believes creative skills are hardwired in people.

"Alzheimer's doesn't usually affect the occipital lobe in the brain, which processes color," Julie explains. "The amygdala, which houses emotional memory, is also hardly impacted by the disease. So people with advanced dementia can appreciate color and feel an emotional connection to something they see."

"I've never met someone who is not creative,
who could not enjoy some art form."

One of Julie's specialties is making murals that help elders tell the stories of their lives through art. Though her larger pieces may include as many as 200 people, she does most of her work one-on-one, interviewing individuals and involving each person in the creation and in the painting process.

"So people with advanced dementia can appreciate color and feel an emotional connection to something they see."

Draw Out a Story

"Care partners can easily adapt my techniques to capture key parts of their lives in a drawing or painting," says Julie.

You just need to be willing to explore and experiment. For those who don't feel comfortable drawing, Julie suggests using tracing paper so you can outline stencils or pictures in magazines or books. You can also find clip art online. Or photocopy a favorite family photo, enlarge it, then trace around it so you can paint within that outline.

Weaving together these life stories and sketches can be an ongoing project, depicting family heritage, life interests, and accomplishments. You can invite others to join in. Julie suggests having art supplies easily available, so when your partner becomes bored or restless, you can quickly turn to painting.

Julie says, "I never ask, 'Dorothy, will you come and paint with me?' I say, 'Dorothy, I have to make a decision and I need your help. I can't think of what color to use. Can you help me?'"

Usually, people are eager to offer advice.

"A red would look nice there," Dorothy might say.

Julie puts some red on a brush, hands it over, and soon Dorothy is painting away.

"People often say, 'I can't do this, I'm not artistic,'" Julie says. "But once I hand them the paintbrush, they're engaged."

Creative Sparks

★ Discuss favorite pets, people, objects, and accomplishments your partner would like to include in a life-story painting.

★ Outline the drawing by sketching, tracing, or downloading line art. Or ask an artistic friend to help.

★ Use water-based acrylic paints; the colors are brilliant and they dry quickly.

★ Sit down and start painting together. For reluctant artists, ask for help choosing a color. For those who need assistance getting started, invite them to select a color and put the paint on the brush for them. Offer encouragement and support as needed.

★ Let the drawing process bring out conversation and use open-ended questions to keep the discussion flowing.

Weave In Fabric

"Through witnessing each other's artwork we are able to witness each other's presence in the world. Through stitching seams or creating felted objects together we also make our relationships stronger. In painting or drawing collaboratively we reach out and touch the marks made by our neighbors, stretching out of our often closely-contained borders." —Caroline Edasis

Maddy paced around the table during the handloom-weaving project. While others participated in group activities, it was often hard to persuade Maddy to sit at the table. Art therapist Caroline Edasis, who facilitated the project, observed that Maddy was restless. Then an aide mentioned that Maddy used to be a home economics teacher. Of course, when it came to sewing-oriented projects, the teacher would be walking around the table, checking on everyone's work. Caroline invited Maddy to accompany her, in observing and assisting others, and Maddy happily took up her old role.

"Creative projects provide wonderful opportunities for connection. They offer a level playing field and don't require a traditional conversation," says Caroline, a multimedia artist and art therapist and Manager of Art Therapy at Mather LifeWays in Evanston, Illinois. "Even people who never identified as artists can really tap into their innate ability."

"Creative projects provide wonderful opportunities for connection. They offer a level playing field and don't require a traditional conversation."

Caroline often encourages fiber arts because they are tactile, easy to use, and easy to connect with an individual's unique life story. She imbues each session with meaning by asking herself such questions as, "How can working with art materials also build connections? What is the therapeutic goal of our time together?"

A Good Yarn and Heartfelt

> "It's important to create, and making art gives people a voice so they can express who they are."

Initially, Caroline tries to learn about people's relationships with fabrics. What materials are they familiar with? Do they have experience mending clothes, weaving, or crocheting? What are their preferred fabrics, textures, and colors? She tailors each project to the participants' interests, abilities, and emotional needs.

For many, there's a comforting rhythm in repetitive activities, such as weaving and felting.

"Interacting with wool is a rich tactile and sensory experience," Caroline says. "Even if your partner is not involved in the weaving, she can touch the wool, sort the colors, wrap the wool around something, or form a playful pattern with the yarn."

For a relaxing activity, Caroline recommends wrapping colorful yarn around an old frame or even a tree branch. She also puts together a simple loom by making evenly spaced notches on the short sides of a picture frame then stringing yarn through those notches, so it's stretched the length of the frame. She can then guide people to weave varying colors of yarn over-and-under, making a small decorative "rug" or wall hanging. Those who don't care for weaving often enjoy tying together fabric strips and rolling them into a ball.

Felting involves putting roving wool (before it's spun into yarn) into warm soapy water, teasing apart the wool, then rolling the wool to make shapes. In this soothing enterprise, you and your partner can form flowers, animals, balls, or other shapes and objects then let them air-dry.

"When you are living with dementia, it can be hard to hold onto your sense of purpose," Caroline says. "It's important to create, and making art gives people a voice so they can express who they are."

Creative Sparks

★ You don't need to have an interest in sewing to enjoy the sensory experience of working with fabrics.

★ Buy small packets of colorful roving wool for an easy felting project. Take your time pulling apart the strands of wool in warm soapy water. Make free-form objects or wrap wool around pipe cleaners to fashion snakes and flowers.

★ Try relaxing, repetitive activities, such as wrapping yarn around a frame or around a basket handle or weaving with a homemade loom.

Connect through Collage

"Collage is like a hall of mirrors. Every direction you look, you see something different and visually stimulating." —Nita Leland

In the 1990s, Jytte Fogh Lokvig, PhD, found herself in a quandary. She was doing a favor for a friend, visiting the friend's mom weekly while the friend was out of the country for three months. The mom lived in long-term care, and the first visit went well. But the second visit shocked Jytte.

"Her mom started screaming and cursing," Jytte says. "I went to the nurses' station to figure out what was wrong. The nurse told me she had Alzheimer's."

Jytte, who lives in Santa Fe, New Mexico, had experience in art and working with at-risk youth but knew nothing about dementia. At the local library, she found only two books on the subject. She read the first few pages of the classic *The 36-Hour Day*, and thought, *What have I gotten myself into?*

But Jytte was not a woman to shy away from a challenge. Using some of the principles she'd employed with youth, she began offering additional activities for the people who were living with dementia.

"I didn't view people with dementia as sick," she says. "Everything I planned was directed at the well part of the person."

She analyzed the home's activities calendar, which was broken up into sixty-minute slots, and realized that accomplishing something in an hour could be challenging for people living with dementia, who often need plenty of time to orient themselves to new situations. She looked for activities that were collaborative rather than competitive so everyone could bloom with a feeling of accomplishment.

"I started with a group collage," she says. "That way, we were all working together."

The collective energy helped break the ice and encouraged people to participate.

"Engagement and conversation are the important things. If it never gets beyond discussing a picture of daisies reminiscent of her growing up garden, that's fine."

Through the process of creating collectively, people relaxed and became comfortable with the materials. This experience was so fulfilling to participants that Jytte began working with families, guiding them in doing projects together.

Jytte suggests collages because they're easy, and there is no right or wrong.

"Collect old magazines, buy a few glue sticks, and break down big boxes to use for cardboard," she suggests. "Keep it simple; if you buy expensive supplies, you may feel a pressure to succeed. This way, it doesn't matter. Engagement and conversation are the important things. If it never gets beyond discussing a picture of daisies reminiscent of her growing up garden, that's fine."

Jytte believes it's important to allow enough time so people work at their own pace. When possible, invite others to join you for the collage experience. Introduce the project by asking the person with dementia for help, saying, "Hey Mom, I'm really interested in this project. Want to help me?"

"Asking for help puts you on an even level and allows the person living with dementia to feel useful," Jytte says.

Creative Sparks

★ Tear pictures out of art, travel, and other colorful magazines.

★ Let your partner direct the artistic action.

★ Use the pictures to trigger conversation.

★ Allow enough time so no one feels rushed.

★ Enjoy the moment and don't worry about a finished product.

Cut, Paste, and Converse

"Art is the only way to run away without
leaving home." —Twyla Tharp

The hospice art therapist shows up at our house, rolling a suitcase filled with supplies. Her client, my life partner Ron's ninety-seven-year-old mother, Mollie, is slumped on our sofa, her head thrown back, her eyes closed.

"Hi Mollie. I'm Denise, the art therapist." Denise introduces herself, even though they have met several times.

"Whatever," Mollie says.

Denise unzips her suitcase and begins taking out art supplies—pink, red, yellow, and green bolts of crunchy tissue paper; a plastic box of small, colorful felt squares, hearts, circles, stars, and triangles; two bottles of Mod Podge glue; and several paint brushes.

Denise settles beside Mollie with a black piece of paper and some red and pink tissue.

"What color do you like best?" she asks.

Mollie shrugs but points to the pink. Denise paints a strip of glue onto her paper and sticks on a crumpled bud of rose-colored paper.

"Mollie, what shape appeals to you?" Denise asks, offering a purple felt square and a red triangle.

Mollie points to the square, then says, "I don't know what to do"—a frequent refrain. Her encroaching confusion has knocked the center out of her normal confidence and rendered her nervous.

"Just sit here with me and help me make this picture," Denise says. Denise offers Mollie a choice between lilac and purple tissue, then sea green and dark green.

"You're an artist," Mollie says, looking at the tissue flowers that have miraculously bloomed on the page. A garden is beginning. "You're really an artist," Mollie repeats.

Denise smiles. "Thank you Mollie. Can you take this brush and spread the glue?"

The brush shakes in Mollie's hand, but she manages to even out the glue, preparing the page for a tangerine and lemon colored blossom.

"This is art," Mollie says.

"You like art, don't you?" Denise says. "You have quite an art collection."

Mollie nods. As she spreads the next glob of glue, Denise asks her about the antique shop she ran for many years and her travels to purchase art. Mollie answers, but she seems more focused on the page in front of her, the new art that Denise is bringing into her life.

Creative Sparks

★ When working on an art project together, select bright and appealing colors.

★ Offer opportunities to make choices, such as between blue or red or between a heart shape and a star shape.

★ Include relaxing and easy actions, such as tearing, gluing, or choosing pictures.

★ Create an easily recognizable object, such as a flower, heart, or tree.

★ Use the process to encourage reminiscence and conversation.

CHAPTER ELEVEN

Dive into Playfulness, Games, Fiddling, and Technology

Play On

Invite Playfulness

Dig into Delightfully Destructive Dominoes

Keep a Pocket Full of Memories

Forage in a Fiddle Box

Plug into Technology to Connect

Play On

"We don't stop playing because we grow old; we grow old because we stop playing!" —George Bernard Shaw

When my mother Fran was barely a teenager, she suffered a double loss that squashed her playful spirit. It was the mid-1930s, and thirteen-year-old Fran sat on the boarding house steps, looking mournfully down the street and wondering if her father would really come back for her, as he'd promised. Her mother had recently died, and her father, flung into grief, had thrown up his hands, plunked his daughter in a boarding house, and disappeared.

He did eventually return, but those months of sadness, anxiety, and abandonment took their toll on my mother. Her sense of playfulness dissipated, peeking out only on special occasions.

Dementia allowed my mother's sense of childlike wonder to emerge and blossom. She loved silly faces, odd sounds, and cheerful accessories. She loved to rummage through purses, pockets, and containers.

"Play reinvigorates the body, expands the
mind, and refreshes the spirit."

My life partner Ron's mother, Mollie, was a caretaker for her ailing mother when she was a teen. She too grew up serious, a practical and smart woman. She loved to play cards, games of chance, and embraced the computer in her later years. Even when Mollie no longer knew the time of day, she could still win at Bingo.

Even after a dormant spell, our sense of play can return.

"Play is an unfettering of mind and body," says author, poet, and Funshop creator John Killick. "It calls upon hidden reserves of humor. Play reinvigorates the body, expands the mind, and refreshes the spirit."

Have fun rummaging around in this chapter for easy and playful activities. You'll discover tips to enliven your afternoon cup of coffee and uncover ideas for games that can spark communications. You'll see how technology can keep your family connected and creative and learn how to readily adapt leading edge ideas into hours of play and pleasure.

Invite Playfulness

"The creation of something new is not accomplished by
the intellect but by the play instinct." — Carl Jung

Creativity, imagination, and dreams make life worthwhile, Claire Craig, PhD believes.

She facilitated a session in a memory unit where everyone talked about their hopes and dreams.

"I would like to have tea with the Queen," Claire told the group.

"I'd live in the old Wild West," one elder said.

"I want to take a long train journey," another said.

"I'm jumping out of an airplane."

With her camera, Claire took a photo of each dreamer and later photoshopped the picture into their dream situation. When they met again, they saw themselves as cowboys, train riders, and airplane jumpers. Claire was there as well, sipping tea with her majesty.

"People with a dementia diagnosis don't often get to talk about their dreams."

Claire says. "This exercise encourages them to think wide, and it can also inspire a deep conversation."

Creativity, imagination, and dreams make life
worthwhile, Claire Craig, PhD believes.

Play Dates

> Sprinkling play through daily life is like adding dark chocolate frosting to a plain vanilla cupcake.

Claire Craig and John Killick are coauthors of the book *Creativity and Communication in Persons with Dementia.*

"With a diagnosis of dementia, you can concentrate on the losses or you can focus on the opportunities," John says. "Playfulness is an opportunity that can emerge with dementia."

Sprinkling play through daily life is like adding dark chocolate frosting to a plain vanilla cupcake. John rekindled his own sense of playfulness when he created the Funshop gatherings that are all about play. He orchestrated Funshops in memory care units, and families used the ideas at home to invite playful self-expression and laughter.

Here are a few of John's creations, which you can enjoy with your partner.

Blooming Fun: Let your partner know you are going to play. Tell her, "I am sniffing a flower." Then act it out. Let your partner know how marvelous or horrible it smells by your facial expressions. Hand the imaginary flower to your partner and ask her to sniff it. Watch for her reaction. After she hands it back, take an exaggerated sniff and pretend you've just smelled a skunk. Act out the awful smell and invite her to take a quick whiff.

Giggle Goads: Try to make each other laugh without touching and without words. To get the giggles going, make a silly face, imitate an animal, make an unusual sound, or perform an odd gesture.

Mirror Images: Ask your partner to move his arms. Stand in front of him and mimic his motions. Then ask him to imitate your gestures. "In this nonverbal game, you and your partner must pay close attention to body language and movement," John says.

Chitter-Chatter: Try to convince each other of something by using nonsense syllables. This playful game releases both of you from the confines of words and encourages exaggerated gestures and expressions.

Chocolate Monday and Blue Tuesday

"Transforming a routine into a special
event sparks peoples' imaginations."

"Creativity is about doing something ordinary in a different way," Claire says. "Transforming a routine into a special event sparks peoples' imaginations."

To begin jazzing up everyday activities, Claire invites families to try these suggestions:

- Transform afternoon tea/coffee time.
- Offer a choice of teas, coffees, or even waters.
- Select an interesting cup or mug.
- Add sugar lumps instead of granulated.
- Serve a fruit or sweet with the beverage.
- Put on a hat or scarf for the occasion.
- Play background music.
- Invite a family member or friend to join you.

Theme for a Day

Toss in a theme day and involve family and friends, for example:

- Chocolate Day (or pick a flavor you both enjoy)—How much chocolate can you get?
- Blue Day—Enjoy blue clothes, blue foods, the blues, and more.

- Photo Day—Focus your lens on shooting pictures or looking at photos.
- Art Day—Leaf through art books and create a little art of your own.

It's Official: You Have Permission to Have Fun

> "But creative play is a necessity, not a luxury."

Claire often talks to care partners about well-being, releasing tension, and getting in touch with what's important to them.

"As a care partner, you need to give yourself permission to have fun and play," Claire tells them. "We can become locked into safety and health issues. But creative play is a necessity, not a luxury."

During these discussions, people living with dementia will often chime in and say to their care partner, "Claire's right. That's what I've been telling you."

Creative Sparks

★ Schedule daily creative time on your calendar.

★ Be curious and don't expect a certain outcome. The playful activities will be different each time.

★ Use John Killick's Funshop ideas to enhance your creative connection. Pretend to smell a flower. Chatter earnestly away in gibberish. Top off your playful persona with a straw hat, beret, tam, winter ski cap, or old-fashioned bonnet.

★ Add something unique into an ordinary day. Vary a mealtime routine. Create themed days. For example, celebrate Flower Friday by arranging favorite blossoms, pressing flowers, trying various fragrances, taking a trip to a garden or plant nursery, looking at famous garden paintings, or drawing a still life of various buds and blooms.

Dig into Delightfully Destructive Dominoes

"Play is the beginning of knowledge." — George Dorsey

How can people living with dementia exert some control over their lives?

Eleanor Feldman Barbera, PhD, author of *The Savvy Resident's Guide,* has a theory: a domino theory.

"When you have dementia, you deal with so many frustrations," says Eleanor. "It's difficult to find ways to express these irritations constructively. Dominoes allow a little rebellion within the framework of normal healthy behavior."

The rebellion starts in a low-key way. Eleanor and Annette, a resident of the memory care community, sit at a card table and slowly, and carefully stand up the dominoes. Each one is vertical and is close enough to its neighbor to knock it down with a push. Eleanor moves slowly, letting Annette do most of the work. Annette concentrates as she creates a circle of dominoes that takes over the tabletop. Then, when the loop is complete, Eleanor nods, and Annette nudges the first tile. There is a satisfying crashing sound as the dominoes dramatically tumble, one after another.

"You get to create and destroy within the context of a game," Eleanor says. "This helps release anger and frustration. It's quite cathartic."

Creative Sparks

★ Play Jenga™, where you pull out blocks in a tower, hoping it won't collapse. Or maybe you're secretly hoping it will crash onto the floor.

★ Create a form or object with nontoxic clay then smash it.

★ Build a tower using blocks or playing cards. Once the edifice is tall enough, joyously knock it into oblivion.

Keep a Pocket Full of Memories

"May your pockets be heavy and your heart be light. May good luck pursue you each morning and night." —Irish Blessing

Some memory care residents were slumped in chairs. Others drooped on sofas, their expressions vacant. Others simply lay in bed. When Cathy Treadaway, PhD, received a grant to research play and dementia, she observed that people living with advanced dementia frequently had little to do.

"In late stages of dementia, the world beyond the body is less clear. It's important to have activities and objects nearby," Cathy says.

Playfulness boosts well-being (i.e., happiness and health) throughout life.

Cathy is the Professor of Creative Practice at the Cardiff School of Art and Design, Cardiff Metropolitan University, Wales, United Kingdom. Partnering with academics from other United Kingdom universities, she studied ways to enhance well-being in adults through fostering playfulness. She realized that many adults no longer had permission to play, due to the Western work ethic and society's negative view of playfulness. Yet her research showed that "playful play," which focused more on the experience and not on an end result, was more beneficial to well-being than "achievement-oriented play," such as sports, which could be stressful.

Cathy's research found that playfulness boosts well-being (i.e., happiness and health) throughout life. Additional studies show that happy elders live longer, have fewer falls, and require less medication.

Working with art therapists, nurses, elders, family care partners, technology experts, and designers, Cathy developed a template for personalized pockets, blankets, and aprons designed to comfort and engage. These interactive textiles offer tactile experiences through multiple pouches filled with sensory items. Family and professional care partners can easily create such promising pockets.

Plan Your Pocket

When Cathy and her collaborator Gail Kenning, PhD, were invited to run a Hand iPockets Funshop as part of the Maker's Faire in Sydney, Australia, they wanted to raise awareness of dementia through offering a playful and meaningful project. They had a variety of washable, colorful fabric squares for people to decorate. Their only instructions were, "Make the creation interesting to look at and feel, and put something interesting to touch inside."

Cathy suggested simple things to fiddle and play with, such as beads threaded onto ribbon so they can be moved from side to side, securely attached buttons to fiddle with, or a sewn on zipper to move up and down.

"The pockets are less about memory and more about being in the moment," she says.

At the Maker's Faire, people gathered around long tables, decorating their pockets with buttons, appliques, ribbons, scraps of cloth, and sharing stories as they worked.

These fabrics can be made into pockets then sewn onto blankets, aprons, sweaters, or other articles of clothing.

Material Well-Being

"Dad, we're putting together some of your favorite things," Greg's son tells him. "Can you show us which photos you'd like to include?"

Although Greg can no longer speak, he smiles and points to special photographs. His son has already put together his father's history, including favorite songs, lifelong hobbies, and career interests. With that information, Cathy and her team digitally print the photos onto a cloth booklet, which they attach to the blanket, along with a variety of sewn-on pockets. A big leather pocket relates to a leather woodwork apron that he wore when working in the garden shed. Another pocket holds a series of brightly colored silk handkerchiefs tied together to make bunting. These are soft to touch and interesting to pull out from the pocket. In another pocket, stitched fabric flowers evoke memories of walking in the park in summertime. An MP3 player features Greg's favorite songs.

> "These sensory textiles trigger
> creativity as well as soothe and relax
> both the person making them and
> the person they are made for."

A former fisherman from India lost his swallowing reflex and developed a fear of eating. Cathy's team designed an apron made of brightly colored textiles reminiscent of Indian fabric. They sewed on sizeable beads, buttons, and other chunky objects, so he'd have items to fiddle with. A small stuffed fabric fish in a knotted yarn fishing net adorned one corner. One small pocket contained bus and train tickets. Another pocket contained a muslin pouch with securely attached seashells and pebbles. He wore this throughout the day, often touching the brightly colored materials and mementos. The apron seemed to relax him during meal times. Gradually, he regained his swallowing reflex and began to enjoy mealtimes again.

"People living with dementia still remember emotional and sensory experiences," Cathy says. "Rekindling a sensory life memory, like the particular oily aroma and tactile feeling of worn leather from an old workbag, can be comforting."

Cathy has designed dozens of individualized blankets, aprons, and pockets. Even though she has the advantage of a team, you can easily simplify her ideas to make something engaging for your partner.

"Everybody can be creative. Our every day sensory experiences stimulate ideas that feed our imagination," Cathy says. "These sensory textiles trigger creativity as well as soothe and relax both the person making them and the person they are made for."

Creative Sparks

★ Consider a person's life story when looking for ideas.

★ Consult your partner, offering choices of fabrics, objects, photos, and more. Have fun choosing artifacts that will intrigue your partner.

★ Choose fabrics you can easily wash and dry.

★ Invite others to join you for a pocket party, creating a chance to share stories and ideas. To make a pouch, sew together two fabric squares, leaving one end open. It's important that the sewing is strong and the mementos are attached safely. Attach your pocket creations to a favorite blanket, sweater, or apron using needle and thread. Or use them individually for sensory exploration.

Forage in a Fiddle Box

"It is a happy talent to know how to
play." —Ralph Waldo Emerson

My father is in the kitchen, pouring coffee, and putting cookies on a plate. Mom sits on the sofa, organizing the mail. She stacks the serious business-sized white envelopes then leafs through them one by one, making a new stack on the coffee table. After methodically sifting through again, she carries the pile toward the bathroom.

"Where is Mom taking the mail?" I ask Dad. They've only been in this retirement community for a month, and Dad seems more relaxed in the modest space. It's easier to keep track of Mom.

"Either to the bathroom or the linen closet," he says, handing me the cookies. "It's just junk mail, but she really seems to enjoy carrying it around."

"Fran," Dad says. "Come on in. We're going to have some cookies."

Minutes later, Mom comes in, carrying a few envelopes. "We have so much mail," she tells me.

Intuitively, my father has come up with a free-form version of a playful Fiddle Box. As usual, Dad is thinking outside the box.

Fiddle Fun

"Use fiddle boxes when your partner is restless, anxious, or pacing," Jytte Lokvig, PhD, author of *The Alzheimer's Creativity Project* says. "You can ask for help in sorting and tidying the box."

"Put in stuff you can count, organize, sort,
rearrange, admire, discuss, or simply touch."

Jytte suggests a shoebox or a bigger plastic container, something that's easy to carry. The box needs to look messy and interesting without seeming overwhelming.

"Put in stuff you can count, organize, sort, rearrange, admire, discuss, or simply touch," Jytte says. "You can focus on a theme, such as old watches or baking paraphernalia. Or you can present a potpourri of items."

The objects can tie into the person's hobbies or passions or just be intriguing odds and ends.

Theme Therapy

Tom and Karen Brenner, authors of *You Say Goodbye and We Say Hello*, often help families put together themed boxes. Depending on the partners' interests, families offer collections of ribbons, keys, photos, bits of pipe or hardware items, various size paintbrushes, cookie cutters, and measuring spoons.

"The point is to engage in a variety of tactile experiences," Karen says. "The items are catalysts for connecting."

Tom and Karen try to honor the Montessori principle of using natural, beautiful, and well-kept objects.

Here's one example of how a fiddle box, tray, or bag can engage. Lena was a seamstress and has always loved fabric. She still loves sorting through a tray of beautiful squares of all different cloths. The texture of silk brings up a story about a favorite blue scarf. The rough wool reminds her of her father's old Army blanket, and a swatch of corduroy makes her think of the forest green overalls she made for her daughter's eighth birthday. There are two squares of each fabric, and she likes to sit with her son and grandson and match the different materials. Even though she can't see all the different colors, she discerns the textures, and her ten-year-old grandson is learning about material.

Creative Sparks

★ Make a list of the person's previous passions.

★ Stroll around your house and collect some odds and ends that might intrigue them.

★ Find a shoebox or plastic container that's easy to carry around. Or use a satchel, tray, or mat.

★ Omit anything that can lead to choking or cutting.

★ Include items that are pleasing to touch and interesting to sort, such as office supplies, gardening mementos, baseball cards, postcards, and cooking supplies.

Plug into Technology to Connect

"Any sufficiently advanced technology is
indistinguishable from magic."—Arthur C. Clarke

"Hi Berta, what shall we do today? Want to watch fireworks? Or tour the Louvre? Or visit with your sister in Ames?"

Though Berta is sitting quietly in a wheelchair in a Nebraska memory care household, Cameo Rogers knows that with a click of technology, she and Berta can enjoy any of these options.

A small study has shown that using technology may foster more interaction between relatives and people living with dementia. As a Life Enrichment Coordinator and Certified Therapeutic Recreation Specialist with Vetter Health Services, Cameo has used simple and inexpensive apps, which are simple software programs focused on art, pottery, games, music, and so on, to enliven the horizons of those living with dementia. Family care partners can easily replicate her ideas.

Approach Life Interests through Apps

"Using apps can simplify the artistic process and be a bridge to a person's interests."

Italian dinner music plays in the background. Ernesto touches the computer screen, igniting an explosion of color. He croons along in Italian as he creates a Jackson Pollock style painting on the computer. Before Cameo discovered the painting program, Ernesto, formerly a brilliant artist, had shunned the brush and canvas. His dementia was advancing, and he was verbally aggressive. But reconnecting with art changed Ernesto's behavior and brightened his spirits.

"Using apps can simplify the artistic process and be a bridge to a person's interests," Cameo says. "Residents really respond when they can move their fingers around on a computer screen and create color and designs."

Working one-on-one, Cameo may try a pottery or painting app with residents. Based on their responses, she decides if she wants to try the project with real materials or if the virtual experience is easier and more satisfying.

For example, the *Let's Create Pottery* app simulates shaping clay on a pottery wheel. By touching the screen, people can mold clay, altering size and shape. They can fire, paint, and decorate it, and even sell their art at a simulated auction. The process is rich with choices and chances for conversation.

"Once people get used to touching the screen, they enjoy these activities," Cameo says. She often looks for inspiration and projects by searching creative online sites that allow for sharing images and ideas, such as Pinterest.

Slide into Memories

Cameo clicks her computer mouse, and an adorable baby beams from the screen. Ninety-year-old Agnes beams back then giggles. She loves babies and says, "Oooh, there you are," to the next slide of a chubby one-year-old, licking frosting off a spoon. It's her first smile in a week, and the nurse dabs at a tear. Agnes is in the later stage of dementia and has been withdrawn and depressed. But these images speak to her.

Using technology, Cameo has designed a variety of slide shows for her residents, including a montage featuring wedding dresses, tractors, pets, and flowers. She can show these to groups using a big screen or tailor the presentation for an individual by using her laptop.

"You just need simple pictures and a topic that makes their creative juices flow," she advises.

Share with Family and Friends

"Video conferences have been amazing for us," Cameo says.

Here's one example of Skype's videoconferencing magic:

Nellie is ninety-seven and living in a memory care household in eastern Nebraska. Her sister, Velma, is ninety-five and lives in a care community in central Nebraska. They haven't seen each other in years.

Until Skype, that is. The care staff and their children facilitate the call so the sisters can talk. They are thoroughly engaged and animated during the conversation, thrilled to be connected.

Cameo encourages people living with dementia and their families to use Skype to stay connected with friends and relatives and to virtually attend important family occasions, such as weddings, bridal showers, birthday parties, and holiday celebrations. Skype also allows residents to watch their grandchildren play or perform.

"Connect during a time when everyone is well-rested," she suggests. "Make the experience short and non-threatening, without any pressure to talk or answer questions."

View Videos as Teachers

Targeted videos offer another chance for sensory engagement. Residents may hold rolling pins, pie tins, or spatulas while watching a video about making an apple pie. Then they talk about the baking process and share personal stories. They can also use the video instructions to actually make a pie.

Use Technology to Strengthen Ties

Jack York understands how transformative the right combination of technology and personal interests can be. Jack left a lucrative career in Silicon Valley to found It's Never 2 Late (iN2L). His company creates software programs for care facilities that allow families and staff to integrate the residents' interests with various games and artistic projects. He encourages family care partners to use his ideas at home.

He recommends Google Earth as a wonderful tool to reminisce and see the world. With the downloadable program, you can revisit a childhood street (Warning: It might not look the same), travel the Nile, or look at the beach where the family used to vacation. He invites people to search sites that tie into their favorite newspapers, magazines, or museums. To view free clips of old movies, classic TV series, comedy sketches, cartoons, songs, and much more, explore YouTube.

"According to our research, technology tailored to those living with dementia considerably improves their quality of life and helps their care partners support the person's unique strengths," Jack says.

Creative Sparks

★ Look for computer applications and ideas that complement your partner's interests and history by searching online or ask friends and relatives for tips. If you have children or grandchildren, get them involved by inviting them to research apps.

★ Search social media sharing sites for ideas on technology and dementia.

★ Issue a low-key invitation, such as "Want to take a look at this map?" Then pause, pointing out and commenting on areas of interest, such as, "There's your son's house."

★ Search for or create simple videos that tap into life skills, such as cake baking, dairy farming, and horseback riding.

★ Use Skype and other video services to connect with friends and family.

ABOUT DEBORAH

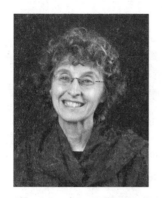Deborah Shouse is a writer, speaker, editor, creativity catalyst, and dementia advocate. She has an MBA but uses it only in emergencies. Her writing has appeared in a variety of publications including the *Washington Post*, *Huffington Post*, *Natural Awakenings*, *Reader's Digest*, *Newsweek*, *Woman's Day*, *Spirituality & Health*, the *Chicago Tribune*, and *Unity Magazine*. Deborah has been featured in many anthologies, including more than four-dozen *Chicken Soup* books. She has written a number of business books, including *Breaking the Ice*, *Nametags Plus*, *Communicating with Difficult People*, and *Marketing Yourself at Work*. For years Deborah wrote a love story column for the *Kansas City Star*.

Deborah initially self-published her book, *Love in the Land of Dementia: Finding Hope in the Caregiver's Journey*. Using the book as a catalyst, Deborah and her partner Ron raised more than $80,000 for dementia programs. Central Recovery Press has published an updated version of this book.

Deborah and Ron have orchestrated workshops and performed her dramatized stories for Alzheimer's Associations and care partners' groups in the United States, New Zealand, Canada, Puerto Rico, England, Ireland, Chile, Costa Rica, Italy, Turkey, and the US Virgin Islands. They have worked with spiritual groups, hospice, healthcare professionals, activity directors, long-term care centers, social workers, and book clubs. Through sharing their message of finding creativity and hope in the dementia journey, they have connected with care partners around the world.

"The person living with Alzheimer's is the pupil in God's eye," a priest in Florence, Italy, told them after one of their performances.

"Your story is my story," a man in Istanbul, Turkey, said.

"When I left home this morning, I was so tired of caring for my husband," a woman from Brooklyn, New York said. "But after hearing your stories, I can once again feel my deep love for him."

To learn more about Deborah's work, visit her blog at DementiaJourney.org. And to share your ideas and stories, please contact Deborah at myinfo@pobox.com

ACKNOWLEDGMENTS

Every writer needs a cheerleader. I was lucky: my cheerleader lives right on location. My life partner, Ron Zoglin, offered encouragement around the clock as needed. He read every section of the book many times and then read the entire book out loud to me. He was supportive, enthusiastic, and always insightful. He turned our home into a writer's retreat, often cooking me a "writer's omelet" and delivering the occasional boost of dark chocolate. I cannot thank him enough.

My family helped keep me grounded and connected during my writing process. I am so grateful for their energy, humor, and sweet presence.

I am lucky to be surrounded by wonderful writers, editors, friends, and colleagues.

My weekly critique partners, Andrea Warren and Barbara Bartocci, offered me astute edits, discerning writing advice, and steadying support throughout the process. They helped me shape the book and critiqued every chapter, often multiple times. I am so grateful for their unwavering assistance. My novel-writing critique group understood when I abandoned my fiction and plunged into this book. Judith Fertig, Jacqueline Guidry, Linda Rodriguez, and Robin Silverman read, critiqued, and offered me vital advice and insights.

Maril Crabtree reviewed the chapters from both an editor's and a care partner's viewpoint and helped me stay focused and inspired. Susan Fenner was wonderfully enthusiastic while giving me smart and practical suggestions. Carmen Mendieta offered compassionate guidance and grounding.

When I started the project, my friend, poet, and editor Candy Schock said, "I will help you in any way I can." She helped in innumerable ways, including doing research, giving me feedback on the full manuscript, and helping me get organized, a daunting task at best.

I reached out to a variety of people, asking for feedback on various chapters. They helped me further fine tune the book so it could be useful to care partners. A heartfelt thank you to Betty Barnett, Jennie Burt, Liz Campbell, Barbara Dooley, Michael Duffy, Catherine Goodson, Mary-Lane Kamberg, Sandra Kinney, Kelly Loeb, Johnna Lowther, Carmen Mendieta, Elizabeth Miller, Teri Miller, Michelle Niedens, Sarah Grace Parlak, Jackie Pinkowitz, Terrill Petri, Clemme Rambo, Jeanne Reeder, Mandy Shoemaker, Hilee Shouse, Sarah Shouse, Carol Smith, Suzanne Smith, Bernadette and Ed Stankard, Vicki Stoecklin, Barbara Unell, Kay Wallack, and Suzanne Willey. I am so grateful for their insights and their generosity of spirit and heart.

The Kansas City Writers Group is a constant source of inspiration, and I am blessed by their presence in my life. Thanks to my agent, Regina Ryan, for her patient direction. I am delighted to be working with the team at Central Recovery Press again. Many of them have experience as care partners, and they are passionate advocates for those living with dementia. All of them were accessible, willing to offer assistance as needed, and enthusiastic about the book.

My humble and heartfelt thanks goes to my contributors. Each of them inspired me and enriched my life. I hope their stories and ideas will enrich yours.

ABOUT THE
CONTRIBUTORS

Ariadne (Ari) Albright, MFA, is the Arts Program Coordinator and Artist in Residence for Sanford Vermillion Medical Center in Vermillion, SD. As a roster artist with the South Dakota Arts Council's Artists in the Schools and Communities Program since 2007, Ari's specialization has become arts engagement in healthcare environments. www.arialbright.com

Eleanor Feldman Barbera, PhD, is an accomplished speaker, eldercare coach, and consultant with nearly twenty years of experience as a psychologist in long-term care. She's the award-winning author of *The Savvy Resident's Guide* and McKnight's LTC News column, The World According to Dr. El. She writes extensively about mental health issues in LTC. www.Eldercarewithdrel.com

Anne Basting, PhD, is an educator, scholar, playwright, speaker, and artist. She has developed and researched methods for embedding the arts into long-term care, with a focus on people with cognitive disabilities like dementia. She is founder and President of the award-winning TimeSlips Creative Storytelling, which replaces the pressure to remember with the freedom of imagination. www.TimeSlips.org

Laura Beck has worked for The Eden Alternative, an international, non-profit focused on creating quality of life for Elders and their care partners since 2003. Her personal journey with her late parents inspires her commitment to change the culture of care through the creation of supportive, inclusive, caring communities. www.edenalt.org

Michael Berg serves as an activities director and life enhancement specialist at Highgate Senior Living. His eclectic background includes acting, teaching, writing, comedy, movement, theatre, mime, animal studies, exercise psychology, martial arts, European clowning, sports, yoga, dance, improvisation, stress management, brain-gym awareness, technology, dementia/Alzheimer's services, and memory care.

Erin Bonitto, founder of Gemini Consulting, Life Enrichment Systems for Dementia, is a sought-after speaker and dementia educator who provides dementia communication coaching in professional care settings across the country. Erin is passionate about bringing dementia skill coaching to family and community care partners to ensure they can create meaningful connections with their loved one. www.Gemini-Consulting.org

Mara Botonis's life and career trajectory was forever changed after thirty years in healthcare, when a close family member was diagnosed with Alzheimer's. Her everyday work at the national level alongside countless dementia care professionals and families impacted by Alzheimer's offered her unparalleled opportunities to learn from their collective expertise. She is the author of the book, *When Caring Takes Courage*. whencaringtakescourage.com

Tom Brenner is a gerontologist who specializes in creating dementia care programs that are strength-based and positive leaning. His wife, Karen, is a Montessori educator who cofounded a Montessori school for children who are deaf. The Brenners have worked together for the past twenty years researching and implementing the application of the Montessori Method for positive dementia care. Tom and Karen travel throughout the United States presenting workshops, training programs, and speaking engagements about their uplifting and positive approach to dementia care.

Denise Brown is currently an Art Therapist at Kansas City Hospice in Kansas City, Missouri. She has served in this role for ten years and recently added Grief Support Specialist to her position. Previously, she provided art education in public schools. She loves using art to enhance people's lives.

Jeffrey Burns, MD, MS, is the Edward H. Hashinger Professor of Neurology and Codirector of the Kansas University Alzheimer's Disease Center. He also directs the Frontiers Clinical and Translational Science Unit. Dr. Burns is researching the impact of exercise on the brain, with a goal of learning how to prevent, delay, or slow the advance of dementia.

Cameron J. Camp, PhD, is Director of Research and Development at the Center for Applied Research in Dementia. He is a Fellow and past-president of Division 20 (Adult Development and Aging) of the American Psychological Association. His research has been funded by the National Institutes of Health and the Alzheimer's Association. www.cen4ard.com

Deb Campbell is Founder and Executive Director of Kansas City Senior Theatre and Arts and AGEing KC. She is an entrepreneur with over thirty-five years experience in the field of aging. Deb is an adjunct professor in social gerontology at Benedictine College and specializes in creative aging and drama therapy programming. www.kcseniortheatre.org

Carmela Carlyle is a psychotherapist, Eldercare Specialist, Certified Laughter Yoga Teacher, and Certified Integrative Yoga Therapist. Her DVD, *Laughter Yoga with Older Adults: Joyful Chair Fitness,* is used all over the world. www.carmelacarlyle.com

Garuth Chalfont, PhD, provides design, training, interventions, and research for dementia care environments. Through Dementia Beat Camp® he promotes prevention and non-pharmacological treatments. Garuth is a health researcher at Lancaster University, a Fellow of the Royal Geographical Society, a published author and illustrator, landscape architect, and classically trained percussionist. www.chalfontdesign.com

Karen Clond, LMSW, came to the Alzheimer's Association Heart of America Chapter in 2006. She is the coordinator for the Chapter's Memories in the Making© watercolor art program and also works as a Dementia Care Specialist with individuals and families faced with the challenges of Alzheimer's and related dementias.

Dan Cohen, MSW, is founder and Executive Director of MUSIC & MEMORY[SM], a nonprofit that promotes the use of personalized music to improve the lives of the elderly and infirm. *Alive Inside: A Story of Music & Memory,* a Sundance Audience Award-winning documentary, tells its inspirational story. Music & Memory now operates in thousands of long-term care communities globally. www.musicandmemory.org

Lori Condict is a Regional Lifestyle Consultant with Americare who is very passionate about her residents and her activity programming. She has worked in Adult Day Care and volunteered in several Memory Care communities. She is certified in Dan Cohen's Music & Memory program and is a part of the MC5 Collation for Elders. She loves music and performs Blues and Jazz on the weekends to relax.

Claire Craig teaches occupational therapy specializing in working with older people and people living with dementia. Her research interest includes exploring ways that design can improve the quality of life of older people. She has written and coauthored numerous books and is currently studying for a PhD in participatory photographic research methods in gerontology.

Barbara Dooley enjoys her volunteer work with a number of community organizations including hospice, AARP Tax-Aide, and local performing arts groups. She is a care partner for a relative.

Caroline Edasis is an art therapist in Chicago, Illinois. Her experiences developing arts programs for individuals living with dementia and their caregivers include intergenerational art programs, museum art-viewing, and art-making programs. She works as Manager of Art Therapy for Mather LifeWays in Evanston, Illinois. She also explores themes of aging, memory, and home through her own art practice. www.carolineedasis.com

Charles Farrell, MD, is a retired vascular surgeon and cofounder of the Carolyn L. Farrell Foundation for Brain Health. He created the foundation with his daughter in honor of his wife, Carolyn, who lived with Lewy Body dementia. Charles is a certified TimeSlips™ facilitator, is certified for training in Montessori-based Dementia Programming, and is also a Positive Approach Dementia coach. www.farrellfoundation.com

Judith Fertig maintains that food is another way to tell a story—with a delicious ending. Her best-selling and award-winning cookbooks include *Bake Happy, I Love Cinnamon Rolls!* and *The Back in the Swing Cookbook: Recipes for Eating and Living Well Every Day After Breast Cancer*. Her novels include *The Cake Therapist* and *The Memory of Lemon*. www.judithfertig.com

Suzanne Fitzsimmons, MS, ARNP, TR-C, is a geriatric nurse practitioner and a recreation therapist. She is an instructor in the Department of Gerontology and Recreation Therapy, University of North Carolina at Greensboro, and teaches gerontology for the University of Southern Maine. She has written and lectured extensively on using non-pharmacological interventions for the behavioral and psychological symptoms of dementia.

Judith-Kate Friedman has been named a Distinguished Fellow of the Global Alliance for Arts and Health for her work as founder of Songwriting Works™ and the non-profit Songwriting Works Educational Foundation. She collaborates with communities across the age and health spectrum and performs and teaches internationally. She serves on the National Center for Creative Aging's Speakers and Consultants Bureau. www.songwritingworks.org

Lauren Gaffney decided that after years in business she wanted a job that was more fulfilling. She received a master's degree in occupational therapy in 2012 from Worcester State University. Since then she has been practicing OT with a focus on creating meaning in the lives of individuals living with dementia.

Gary Glazner is the founder and Executive Director of the Alzheimer's Poetry Project (APP). The APP was the recipient of the 2013 Rosalinde Gilbert Innovations in Alzheimer's Disease Caregiving Legacy Award. The APP has worked in twenty-six states and internationally in Australia, Germany, Poland, and South Korea. www.alzpoetry.com

Natasha Goldstein-Levitas, R-DMT, is a Registered Dance/ Movement Therapist with fifteen years of experience working with high functioning to severely cognitively and physically impaired adults and older adults. She incorporates her extensive knowledge of music and vocal artists of the 40s, 50s, 60s and 70s into sessions, along with sensory stimulation techniques.

Cathy Greenblat, PhD, has been engaged in a cross-cultural photographic project on aging, dementia, and end of life care since she retired from Rutgers University. She is Honorary Research Fellow at the International Observatory on End of Life Care, Lancaster University, United Kingdom, and she is the author of *Love, Loss, and Laughter: Seeing Alzheimer's Differently.* www.lovelossandlaughter.com

Kathy Greene joined Silverado in 1998 and is the Senior Vice President of Program and Services Integration for their memory care communities, hospice, and home services. Ms. Greene has worked in long-term care of the elderly for thirty years in a variety of environments, including skilled nursing, assisted living, and county service agencies.

Nathan Hescock, professional dancer and entrepreneur, founded Rhythm Break Productions in 1999, creating a home for other dance professionals to maintain their craft, broaden their ideas, and share their knowledge with others. His non-profit, Rhythm Break Care, is an expression of his knowledge of music, movement, and passion for the elderly community. www.rbcares.org

Berna Huebner is co-director of the film *I Remember Better when I Paint* and editor of the book with the same title. She is president of the Hilgos Foundation and has served on the board of Arts & Minds and on the Boston University Alzheimer's Board. She has been director of the Center of International Communications, Paris, and was Research Director for Governor Nelson Rockefeller. www.hilgos.org and www.irememberwhenipaint.com

Veronica Kaninska, MS Ed, CTRS, has been working with puppets for the past seventeen years. She completed her degree in theater arts in the Ukraine in 1992 and received an honorary diploma. Veronica is a frequent speaker at state conferences where she shares her presentations on how to use puppets as a therapy tool in clinical environments.

Madan Kataria, MD, is the founder of the Laughter Yoga Clubs movement, which started in 1995 in Mumbai, India. Dr. Kataria is an internationally acclaimed speaker and a corporate consultant for holistic health, stress management, teambuilding, leadership, peak performance, and communication skills. He is associated with a number of research projects to measure the benefits of laughter. www.laughteryoga.org

Rebecca Katz, MS, is a nationally recognized wellness chef and nutritional educator. She is the founder of the Healing Kitchens Institute at Commonweal and the author of five cookbooks, including the award winning *Cancer-Fighting Kitchen*, and most recently, *The Healthy Mind Cookbook*. She lives in San Rafael, CA. www.rebeccakatz.com

Tamara Keefe worked for many years as Creative Programming Director, at Elderwise. In this capacity, she enjoyed developing creative engagement opportunities with and for people living with cognitive impairment, and their family and friends. Tamara currently works in Lifelong Recreation for Seattle Parks and Recreation. www.elderwise.org and www.seattle.gov/Parks/Seniors/index.htm

John Killick has worked for twenty-three years with people living with dementia and their care partners, notably as Research Fellow in Communication through the Arts at the University of Stirling. He is currently Poet Mentor at the Courtyard Centre for the Arts in Hereford, England, and Writer in Residence for Alzheimer Scotland. www.dementiapositive.co.uk

Shelley Klammer is a registered counsellor, expressive artist, and a therapeutic art instructor. Shelley has developed art programs for children, the general public, incarcerated youth, adults with acquired brain injuries and developmental disabilities, and for people living with dementia. www.expressiveartworkshops.com

Lori La Bey is a passionate advocate for those living with dementia. She serves as the host of Alzheimer's Speaks Radio and the webinar series Dementia Chats™. Lori connects people to best practices and facilitates conversations regarding needs for dementia care worldwide. Her blog, Alzheimer's Speaks, was recognized as the #1 influencer online for Alzheimer's. www.alzheimersspeaks.com

Jytte Lokvig, PhD, is the author of *The Alzheimer's Creativity Project*. She loves working with the elderly, especially those living with dementia. She coaches families and professional caregivers and designs life-enrichment programs for care-facilities. Lokvig introduced the Alzheimer's Cafe to the US. Her workshops and seminars explore effective communication and promote a healthy environment based on dignity and humor. www.AlzheimersAtoZ.com

Johnna Lowther has worked in senior healthcare since 2001, with an educational background in music and psychology and has a personal passion for serving the person and families affected by dementia. She is Certified Assisted Living Home Operator, Certified Alzheimer's Disease and Dementia Trainer, Certified Dementia Care Manager, and author of *Through the Eyes of Dementia: A Pocket Guide to Caregiving.* www.johnnalowther.com

Marie Marley is the award-winning author of *Come Back Early Today: A Memoir of Love, Alzheimer's and Joy,* and the coauthor (with neurologist Daniel C. Potts, MD) of *Finding Joy in Alzheimer's: New Hope for Caregivers.* She blogs on the Huffington Post and Alzheimer's Reading Room. Visit her at www.ComeBackEarlyToday.com

Karrie Marshall, who has a background in nursing and person-centered counseling, managed a care home and lectured in health and social care before founding Creativity In Care™. She develops and delivers creative learning programs to promote inclusion and joyfulness. Karrie is the author of *Puppetry in Dementia Care: Connecting through Creativity and Joy* and *A Creative Toolkit for Communication in Dementia Care.* www.creativityincare.org

Julie Gross McAdam, PhD, is a gerontologist, an author, and the program director of MAC.ART, a multi-award winning dementia-specific art-as-recreation therapy program. Since 2001, Julie has directed over three thousand artists in aged and community healthcare settings in Australia and North America to create more than thirty large scale permanent communal artworks that depict the life-story experiences of the contributors. www.macart.com.au

Elizabeth Miller is currently developing new interests following her long career as an educator. That experience in education prepared her with the resourcefulness that benefits her as a caregiver for her husband, Charlie Miller. Often, Charlie acts as Elizabeth's sous-chef in the kitchen. They live in Kansas City, Missouri, where they stay engaged in many activities and travel.

Teri Miller is the Early-Stage Program Manager for the Alzheimer's Association-Houston and Southeast Texas Chapter, where she has been employed since 1996. Teri has also served as an adjunct faculty member at Texas Women's University Graduate School of Occupational Therapy, where she co-taught *Issues in Adaptation: Intervention with Alzheimer's Families.*

Stine Moen received her BA in Professional Dance and Pedagogy from the Norwegian College of Dance, specializing in dance and movement counseling. Stine is currently performing with modern dance companies Body Collider Dance, Ruah Inc., Shirdance, and Modern Gypsies. Stine started dancing with Rhythm Break Cares in 2011 and serves on the Board of Directors. www.rbcares.org

Jeff Nachtigall is a multidisciplinary artist, curator, speaker, and social entrepreneur. Through working as a full-time artist-in-residence at an assisted-living facility for eight years, he developed the Open Studio, a model he has successfully replicated throughout Canada and the United States. This inclusive, client-centered strategy challenges traditional clinical approaches and pushes the boundaries of the arts in health care. www.openstudioprojects.com

Linsey Norton served as Program Director for the Alzheimer's Association, Central and Western Kansas Chapter.

Emily Meyer Olschki, MA, MT-BC, has been a board-certified music therapist since 2001, with degrees from the University of Dayton and the University of Missouri-Kansas City. She has worked with clients in adult and pediatric hospice and palliative care, pediatric hospitalization, and with developmental disabilities.

Kate Pierce is a social worker with the Alzheimer's Association-Greater Michigan Chapter. She has worked in the field of aging for over ten years in various capacities including a multidisciplinary memory clinic, residential care, adult day program, and most recently, developing a program for people with developmental disabilities and dementia.

Jackie Pinkowitz, MEd, is Board Chair of CCAL and Co-leader of the Dementia Action Alliance, which focuses on advancing person-centered services and meaningful living for individuals with dementia across our nation. She has served on numerous national collaboratives for policy and research and is a frequent speaker at national aging conferences. www.daanow.org and www.ccal.org

Cameo Rogers received her bachelor's degree in therapeutic recreation from Northwest Missouri State University. She is a Certified Therapeutic Recreational Specialist, Certified Dementia Practitioner, and a Certified Dementia Care Manager. She serves as the Life Enrichment Coordinator for Vetter Health Services.

Magdalena Schamberger is Artistic Director, CEO, and Cofounder of Hearts & Minds, based in Scotland. She has over twenty-five years' experience in performing, directing, and teaching physical theatre and theatre clowning. In 2001 she launched the unique Hearts & Minds Elderflowers program, using the performing arts to improve the quality of life for people with advanced dementia in a health care environment. www.heartsminds.org.uk

Tryn Rose Seley is a musician, photographer, author, and expressive arts facilitator. She loves to interact with people of every age and does so on a regular basis. She leads musical experiences, shares her caregiver book, and writes every day, sometimes on the back of grocery receipts, other times on the world-wide-web. www.caregiverheart.com

Susan Shifrin is the founding director of ARTZ Philadelphia. She is an art historian, a museum educator and curator, and an arts accessibility advocate. She received her PhD in the History of Art from Bryn Mawr College and has worked on the curatorial and education staffs of a number of large and small museums. www.artzphilly.org

Teepa Snow is one of America's leading dementia training specialists. Her occupational therapy career, spanning over thirty-five years in a wide variety of practice settings, led her to develop Positive Approach™ to Care techniques that are used by families and professionals striving to cope with dementia throughout the world. www.teepasnow.com

Marlon I. Sobol, MT-BC, LCAT, is the manager of music therapy programming at Schnurmacher Center for Rehabilitation and Nursing. He is a professional percussionist and bandleader. His work has been featured in *DRUM! Magazine, Preserving Your Memory Magazine,* and in *The Journal News.* www.schnurmacher.org

Karen Stobbe's world changed dramatically when both of her parents were diagnosed with Alzheimer's. She works to make all those involved with Alzheimer's have a better quality of life. www.in-themoment.net

Vicki Stoecklin is a retired educator and designer of children's projects located abroad and in the United States. She loves working on cards, crafts, and jewelry for the women at a local shelter.

Concetta Tomaino D.A., MT-BC, LCAT, is the Executive Director/cofounder of the Institute for Music and Neurologic Function and Senior Vice President for Music Therapy at CenterLight Health System. Dr. Tomaino is internationally known for her research and lectures on the clinical applications of music and neurologic rehabilitation. Her work has been featured in the media, documentaries, and in books on health and healing. www.Musictherapy.imnf.org

Cathy Treadaway, PhD, is Professor of Creative Practice at CARIAD, Cardiff Metropolitan University, Wales, United Kingdom. She is a Fellow of the Royal Society of Arts and a practicing designer, writer, and educator. She is the Principal Investigator on the AHRC funded LAUGH Project for dementia international research. www.cathytreadaway.com

Laura Voth is the Community Programs Coordinator at the Philbrook Museum of Art. She develops and facilitates programming for audiences including children, teens, college students, senior adults, and people with disabilities and dementia. In addition to her museum work she is a working artist currently based out of Tulsa, Oklahoma. www.philbrook.org

Barrick Wilson's wife, Kristi, is in a Wichita care home. Barrick retired from hospital marketing and community relations to be a full-time caregiver for his wife. He is the Fourth Congressional District Ambassador/Advocate for the Central and Western Kansas Alzheimer's Association chapter. Performing with the Newton Ukulele Tunes Society (NUTS) allows Wilson to follow his passion for music.

Jack York is president and cofounder of It's Never 2 Late (iN2L). In 1999, after spending fourteen years in the Silicon Valley, Jack started a gerontechnology company dedicated to helping older adults realize the full benefits of adaptive technology. He is a sought-after speaker on technology as a means to create personalized experiences that engage, connect, and inspire. www.iN2L.com

John Zeisel, PhD, President and cofounder of Hearthstone Alzheimer Care and the I'm Still Here Foundation is author of *I'm Still Here: A New Philosophy of Alzheimer's Care*. Zeisel lectures internationally on non-pharmacologic treatment for Alzheimer's disease, focusing on the therapeutic effects of the arts and music, the way design of the physical residential environment can reduce symptoms, and the role engaging community activities play in improving memory and quality of life. www.TheHearth.org

Sarah Zoutewelle-Morris is an American artist living in Holland. She is a passionate advocate for the importance of art as a transformative force in society. She is currently working with citizens and town council members to encourage a more creative, participatory approach to local government. Sarah is the author of *Chocolate Rain: 100 Ideas for a Creative Approach to Activities in Dementia Care*. www.szoutewelle.wordpress.com

RESOURCES

*This is just a sampling of the rich resources available for
care partners and people living with dementia.*

Books and E-books

August, Yosaif. *Coaching for Caregivers, How to Reach Out Before You
Burn Out.* Yes to Life Publishing, 2013.

Barbera, Eleanor. *The Savvy Resident's Guide: Everything You Wanted to
Know About Your Nursing Home Stay But Were Afraid to Ask.* Psychology
Insights Press, 2012.

Basting, Anne. *Forget Memory: Creating Better Lives for People with
Dementia.* Baltimore: The Johns Hopkins University Press, 2009.

Basting, Anne. *TimeSlips Creativity Journal.* www.timeslips.org/For-
Facilitators/creativity-journals.

Bell, Virginia and David Troxel. *The Best Friends Book of Alzheimer's
Activities, Volume One and Two.* Towson, MD: Health Professions Press,
Inc., 2008.

Bell, Virginia and David Troxel. *A Dignified Life, Revised and
Expanded: The Best Friends™ Approach to Alzheimer's Care: A Guide for
Care Partners.* Baltimore, MD: Health Professions Press, Inc., 2015.

Borrie, Cathie. *The Long Hello: The Other Side of Alzheimer's.*
Nightwing Publications, 2010.

Botonis, Maria. *When Caring Takes Courage: A Compassionate,
Interactive Guide for Alzheimer's and Dementia Caregivers.* Parker, CO:
Outskirts Press, 2014.

Brackey, Jolene. *Creating Moments of Joy for the Person with Alzheimer's or Dementia: A Journal for Caregivers.* West Lafayette, IN: Purdue University Press, 2007.

Brenner, Tom and Karen Brenner, *You Say Goodbye and We Say Hello: The Montessori Method for Positive Dementia Care.* Brenner Pathways, 2012.

Cail, Mary McDaniel. *Alzheimer's: A Crash Course for Friends and Relatives.* Truewind Press, 2013.

Callone, Patricia, et al. *A Caregiver's Guide to Alzheimer's Disease: 300 Tips for Making Life Easier.* New York: Demos Medical Publishing, 2006.

Camp, Cameron. *Montessori–Based Activities for Persons with Dementia.* Beachwood, OH: Myers Research Institute, 2006.

Canfield, Jack, et al. *Chicken Soup for the Caregiver's Soul: Stories to Inspire Caregivers in the Home, Community and the World.* Deerfield Beach, FL: Health Communications, Inc, 2004.

Chalfont, Garuth and Alex Walker. *Dementia Green Care Handbook of Therapeutic Design and Practice*, 2013. FREE download from www. chalfontdesign.com.

Chalfont, Garuth. *Design for Nature in Dementia Care.* Bradford Dementia Group Good Practice Guide. London: Jessica Kingsley Publishers, 2008.

Craig, Claire, *Exploring the Self through Photography: Activities for Use in Group Work.* London: Jessica Kingsley Publishers, 2009.

Doherty, Janice Hoetker. *A Calendar Year of Horticultural Therapy: How Tending Your Garden Can Tend to Your Soul.* Boynton Beach, FL: Lilyflower Publishing, Inc., 2009.

Doraiswamy, P. Murali and Lisa Gwyther. *The Alzheimer's Action Plan: What You Need to Know—and What You Can Do—About Memory Problems, from Prevention to Early Intervention and Care.* New York: St. Martin's Press, 2008.

Dowling, J. R. *Keeping Busy: A Handbook of Activities for Persons with Dementia.* Baltimore: The Johns Hopkins University Press, 1995.

Femia, Elia and Karen Love. *You Can Help Someone Live Fully with Dementia: A Guide for Family and Friends,* FIT Interactive, 2014.

Gawande, Atul, *Being Mortal: Medicine and What Matters in the End.* New York: Metropolitan Books, Henry Holt and Company, LLC, 2014.

Genova, Lisa. *Still Alice.* New York: Simon & Schuster, 2009.

Gilliard, Jane and Mary Marshall, eds. *Fresh Air on My Face: Transforming the Quality of Life for People with Dementia through Contact with the Natural World.* London: Jessica Kingsley Publishers, 2012.

Glazner, Gary. *Dementia Arts: Celebrating Creativity in Elder Care.* Baltimore, MD: Health Professions Press, Inc., 2014.

Glazner, Gary. *Sparking Memories: The Alzheimer's Poetry Project Anthology.* Poem Factory, 2010.

Goyer, Amy. *Juggling Life, Work, and Caregiving.* Washington, DC: AARP, 2015.

Greenblat, Cathy. *Alive with Alzheimer's,* Chicago: University of Chicago Press, 2004.

Greenblat, Cathy, *Love, Loss, and Laughter: Seeing Alzheimer's Differently.* Guilford, CT: Lyons Press, 2012.

Griffin, Randy. *Bird Tales: A Program for Engaging People with Dementia through the Natural World of Birds.* Baltimore, MD: Health Professions Press, Inc., 2013.

Hartley, Carolyn P. and Peter Wong. *The Caregiver's Toolbox*. Lanham, MD: Taylor Trade Publishing, 2015.

Huebner, Berna, ed. *I Remember Better when I Paint: Art and Alzheimer's: Opening Doors, Making Connections*. Glen Echo, MD: Bethesda Communications Group, 2011.

Joltin, Adena, Cameron Camp, et al. *A Different Visit: Activities for Caregivers and Their Loved Ones with Memory Impairments*. Solon, Ohio: Center for Applied Research and Dementia, 2012.

Katz, Rebecca and Mat Edelson. *The Healthy Mind Cookbook: Big-Flavor Recipes to Enhance Brain Function, Mood, Memory, and Mental Clarity*. Ten Speed Press, 2015.

Katz, Rebecca with Mat Edelson. *The Longevity Kitchen, Satisfying Big-Flavor Recipes*. Ten Speed Press, 2013.

Killick, John, and Kate Allen. *Communication and the Care of People with Dementia*. Buckingham, UK: Open University Press, 2002.

Killick, John, with Claire Craig. *Creativity and Communication in Persons with Dementia*. London: Jessica Kingsley Publishers, 2011.

Killick, John. *Dementia Positive: A Handbook Based on Lived Experiences*. Edinburgh: Luath Press, 2014.

Killick, John. *Playfulness and Dementia: A Practical Guide*. London: Jessica Kingsley Publishers, 2012.

Killick, John, and Anne Basting. *The Arts and Dementia Care: A Resource Guide*. Washington, DC: National Center for Creative Aging, 2003.

Klammer, Shelley. *How to Start an Art Program for the Elderly*, e-book. www.expressiveartworkshops.com.

Lokvig, Jytte and John Becker. *Alzheimer's A to Z: A Quick-Reference Guide*. Oakland: New Harbinger Publications, 2004.

Lokvig, Jytte. *Alzheimer's A to Z, Secrets to Successful Caregiving,* Santa Fe, NM: Endless Circle Press, 2003.

Lokvig, Jytte. *The Alzheimer's Creativity Project.* Santa Fe, NM: Endless Circle Press, 2014.

Lokvig, Jytte. *Alzheimer's and Dementia Relationships and Teamwork Handbook.* Santa Fe, NM: Endless Circle Press, 2015.

Lowther, Johnna. *Through the Eyes of Dementia: A Pocket Guide to Caregiving.* Kansas City, MO: JoJo Studio Press, 2014.

Lunden, Joan and Amy Newmark. *Chicken Soup for the Soul: Family Caregivers: 101 Stories of Love, Sacrifice, and Bonding.* Cos Cob, CT: Chicken Soup for the Soul Publishing, LLC, 2012.

Mace, Nancy and Peter Rabins. *The 36-Hour Day: A Family Guide to Caring for People Who Have Alzheimer's Disease, Related Dementias, and Memory Loss.* New York: Grand Central Publishing, 2012.

Marley, Marie. *Come Back Early Today: A Memoir of Love, Alzheimer's and Joy.* Olathe, KS: Joseph Peterson Books, 2011.

Marley, Marie and Daniel C. Potts, MD. *Finding Joy in Alzheimer's: New Hope for Caregivers.* Olathe, KS: Joseph Peterson Books, 2015.

Marshall, Karrie, *A Creative Toolkit for Communication in Dementia Care.* London: Jessica Kingsley Publishers, 2015.

Marshall, Karrie, *Puppetry in Dementia Care: Connecting through Creativity and Joy.* Jessica London: Kingsley Publishers, 2013.

McCurry, Susan. *When a Family Member Has Dementia: Steps to Becoming a Resilient Caregiver.* Santa Barbara: ABC-CLIO, 2006.

Newmark, Amy and Angela Geiger. *Chicken Soup for the Soul: Living with Alzheimer's & Other Dementias: 101 Stories of Caregiving, Coping, and Compassion.* Cos Cob, CT: Chicken Soup for the Soul Publishing, 2014.

Norris, Katie, and Jennifer Brush. *Creative Connections in Dementia Care: Engaging Activities to Enhance Communication*. Baltimore, MD: Health Professions Press, Inc., 2015.

Possell, Rev. Linn and Teepa Snow. *A Heart Full of GEMS*. Positive Approach, LLC, 2015.

Post, Stephen. *The Moral Challenge of Alzheimer's Disease: Ethical Issues from Diagnosis to Dying*. Baltimore, MD: The Johns Hopkins University Press, 2000.

Power, G. Allen. *Dementia beyond Disease: Enhancing Well-Being*. Baltimore, MD: Health Professions Press, Inc., 2014.

Power, G. Allen. *Dementia beyond Drugs: Changing the Culture of Care*. Baltimore, MD: Health Professions Press, Inc., 2010.

Sabbagh, Marwan and Beau MacMillan. *The Alzheimer's Prevention Cookbook: 100 Recipes to Boost Brain Health*. Ten Speed Press, 2012.

Schamberger, M. "Compassionate Clowning: Improving The Quality of Life of People with Dementia." *Providing Compassionate Health Care: Challenges in Policy and Practice*. New York: Routledge (2014): 139–54.

Seley, Tryn. *15 Minutes of Fame: One Photo Does Wonders to Bring You Both Back to Solid Ground*. Sudbury, MA: eBookIt.com, 2013.

Shouse, Deborah. *Love in the Land of Dementia: Finding Hope in the Caregiver's Journey*. Las Vegas, NV: Central Recovery Press, 2013.

Stankard, Bernadette and Amy Viets. *Dancing in the Dark: How to Take Care of Yourself when Someone You Love Is Depressed*. Las Vegas, NV: Central Recovery Press, 2012.

Stettinius, Martha. *Inside the Dementia Epidemic: A Daughter's Memoir*. Horseheads, NY: Dundee-Lakemont Press, 2012.

Swaffer, Kate. What the Hell Happened to My Brain? Living beyond Dementia. Jessica Kingsley Publishers, 2016.

Taylor, Richard. *Alzheimer's from the Inside Out*. Baltimore, MD: Health Professions Press, Inc., 2007.

Thomas, William H. *Life Worth Living: How Someone You Love Can Still Enjoy Life in a Nursing Home*. VanderWyk & Burnham, 1996.

Thomas, William H. *What Are Old People For? How Elders Will Save the World*. St. Louis, MO: VanderWyk & Burnham, 2004.

Wallack, Max and Carolyn Given. *Why Did Grandma Put Her Underwear in the Refrigerator?: An Explanation of Alzheimer's Disease for Children*. CreateSpace, 2013.

Zeisel, John. *I'm Still Here: A New Philosophy of Alzheimer's Care*. New York: Penguin Group, 2009.

Zgola, Jitka. *Doing Things: A Guide to Programming Activities for Persons with Alzheimer's Disease and Related Disorders*. Baltimore, MD: The John's Hopkins University Press, 1987.

Zoutewelle, Sarah. *Chocolate Rain: 100 Ideas for a Creative Approach to Activities in Dementia Care*. London: Hawker Publications, Ltd., 2015.

CDs, DVDs, and Videos

Carlyle, Carmela. *Laughter Yoga with Older Adult*. www.carmelacarlyle.com.

Elderflowers and Clown Doctors. *Hearts & Minds: Behind the Nose*. www.vimeo.com/111185931.

Greenblat, Cathy. Love, Loss & Laughter—Living with Dementia www.youtube.com/watch?v=bUT3qQFWDvw.

Hale, Thomas, Director. *A Year at Sherbrooke*: National Film Board of Canada. Jeff Nachtigall and the origins of Open Studio in long-term care. www.nfb.ca/film/year_at_sherbrooke.

Huebner, Berna and Eric Ellena, Co-directors, *I Remember Better when I Paint: Treating Alzheimer's through the Creative Arts*. DVD. http://www.irememberbetterwhenipaint.com.

Kataria, Madan, MD. *100 Laughter Yoga Exercise Videos*. www.youtube.com/watch?v=Fq4kTZuLops.

Paint Pouring. www.sploid.gizmodo.com/pouring-paint-on-top-of-paint-creates-mind-melting-art-1686208250.

Red Nose Coming. Clowning and dementia in care homes; Dementia Services Development Centre 2009. www.dementiashop.co.uk/products/red-nose-coming-dvd-clowning-and-communication-care-homes.

Rhythmic Activities for Everyday Care. Institute for Music and Neurologic Function, Featuring Tomaino, Concetta, and Sobol, Marlon, sponsored by the New York State Department of Health www.imnf.org/.

Sobol, Marlon, Shem's Disciples, *Keep On Moving*, Audio CD. www.amazon.com/Keep-On-Moving-Marlon-Sobol/dp/B013MQ8HYY.

Snow, Teepa. *Filling the Day with Meaning*, and other meaningful free videos, www.teepasnow.com/.

Websites and Blogs

For information on dementia, care partnering, person-centered care, communications, resources, research, advocacy, improving lives, and more, visit these websites:

Alzheimer's Association. www.alz.org/.

Alzheimer's Disease International. www.alz.co.uk/.

Alzheimer's Foundation of America. www.alzfdn.org/.

Alzheimer's Reading Room. www.alzheimersreadingroom.com/.

Alzheimer's Speaks. www.alzheimersspeaks.com/.

Changing Aging. www.changingaging.org/.

Dementia Spotlight Foundation.
www.dementiaspotlightfoundation.org/.

Eden Alternative. www.edenalt.org/.

My Better Nursing Home. www.eldercareWithDrEl.com/.

National Council of Certified Dementia Practitioners.
www.nccdp.org/cdp.htm.

Positive Approach to Care. www.teepasnow.com/.

Powered by Inspiration. www.mariashriver.com/.

Purple Angel Dementia Awareness Campaign.
www.purpleangel-global.com/.

Puzzles to Remember. www.puzzlestoremember.org/.

When Caring Takes Courage. whencaringtakescourage.com/.

Us Against Alzheimer's. www.usagainstalzheimers.org/.

Validation Training Institute. www.vfvalidation.org/.

For more information on these meaningful creative projects, please visit:

Alzheimer's Cafes. www.AlzheimersAtoZ.com/.

Alzheimer's Poetry Project. www.alzpoetry.com/.

The Art of Improvisation. www.in-themoment.com/.

ARTZ (Artists for Alzheimer's). www.imstillhere.org/artz/.

Caregiver's Voice. www.thecaregiversvoice.com/.

Carolyn L. Farrell Foundation. Bringing art into your life. www.farrellfoundation.com/.

Center for Applied Research in Dementia. A wealth of information and videos for families. www.cen4ard.com/.

Chalfont Design. www.chalfontdesign.com/. Gardening ideas.

Conductorcise®—A Sound Workout for Body and Soul. www.conductorcise.com/.

Creativity in Care. www.creativityincare.org/.

Dementia Journey by Deborah Shouse. Deborah's blog on creativity and dementia. www.dementiajourney.org/.

Dementia Positive. www.dementiapositive.co.uk/.

Expressive Arts Work Shop. www.expressiveartworkshops.com/.

Hands Project. www.handsproject.info/.

Hearts and Minds. www.heartartsminds.org.uk/.

Hilgos Foundation. www.hilgos.org/.

I'm Still Here Foundation. www.imstillhere.org/artz/meet-me-movies/.

Inside the Dementia Epidemic. www.insidedementia.com/.

Institute for Music and Neurological Function. www.musictherapy.imnf.org/.

Laughter Yoga. www.laughteryoga.org/.

Love, Loss and Laughter. www.lovelossandlaughter.com/.

MAC.ART Program Director. www.macart.com.au/.
Dr. Julie Gross McAdam and her fascinating murals that she creates with people who are living with dementia.

Meet Me at MoMa. www.moma.org/meetme/.

Music & Memory. www.musicandmemory.org/.

National Center for Creative Aging. www.creativeaging.org/.

Open Studio Projects. www.openstudioprojects.com/.

Puzzles to Remember. www.puzzlestoremember.org/.

Rhythm Break Cares (RBC) Dance for Dementia programs. www.rbcares.org/

The Society for the Arts in Dementia Care. www.cecd-society.org/.

Songwriting Works™. Judith-Kate Friedman Educational Foundation. www.songwritingworks.org/.

TimeSlips™. www.timeslips.org/.

To learn from people living with dementia, and about advocacy and community building, view:

Creating life with words: Inspiration, love and truth. www.kateswaffer.com/.

Dementia Action Alliance. www.daanow.org/.

Dementia Alliance International. www.dementiaallianceinternational.org/membership/.

Dementia-Friendly Communities. www.actonalz.org/dementia-friendly/.

Scottish Dementia Work Group. www.sdwg.org.uk/useful-links/.

BIBLIOGRAPHY

Allison, Theresa. "Songwriting and transcending institutional boundaries in the nursing home." In *Oxford Handbook of Medical Ethnomusicology*, ed. Ben Koen (Oxford: Oxford University Press, 2008), 240–43.

Ballard, C. et al., "Aromatherapy as a safe and effective treatment for the management of agitation in severe dementia: the results of a double blind, placebo controlled trial." *Journal of Clinical Psychiatry* 63, no. 7 (2002): 553–58.

Chalfont, Garuth E. "Charnley Fold: a practice model of environmental design for enhanced dementia day care." *Social Care and Neurodisability* 2 no. 2 (2011): 71–79.

Chalfont, Garuth E. "The living edge: connection to nature for people with dementia in residential care." In *Understanding Care Homes: A Research and Development Perspective*, eds Katherine Froggatt, Sue Davies, and Julienne Meyer. (London: Jessica Kingsley Publishers, 2008): 109–31.

Cysarz, Dirk, Dietrich von Bonin, Helmut Lackner, Peter Heusser, Maximilian Moser, and Henrik Bettermann. "Oscillations of heart rate and respiration synchronize during poetry recitation." *American Journal of Physiology Heart and Circulatory Physiology* 287, no. 2 (2004): H579–87.

Douglas, Simon, Ian James, and Clive Ballard. "Non-pharmacological interventions in dementia." *Advances in Psychiatric Treatment* 10, no. 3 (2004): 171–77.

Fritsch, T. et al. "Impact of TimeSlips, a Creative Expression Intervention Program, on Nursing Home Residents with Dementia and Their Caregivers." *The Gerontologist* 49, issue 1 (2009): 117–27.

Gerdner, Linda. "Effects of individualized versus classical 'relaxation' music on the frequency of agitation in elderly persons with Alzheimer's disease and related disorders." *International Psychogeriatrics* 12, no. 1 (2000): 49–65.

Kawabata, Hideaki and Semir Zeki. "Neural correlates of beauty." *Journal of Neurophysiology* 91, no. 4 (2004): 1699–1705.

Killick, John and M. Schamberger. "Clowning and connecting: Elderflowers ten years on." *Journal of Dementia Care* 23, no. 1 (2015): 19–21.

Killick, John and Kate Allan. "The arts in dementia care: Tapping a rich resource." *Journal of Dementia Care* 7, issue 4 (1999): 35–38.

King, Abby C. et al. "Moderate-intensity exercise and self-rated quality of sleep in older adults. A randomized controlled trial." *Journal of the American Medical Association* 277, no. 1 (1997): 32–37.

Lord, Thomas R. and Joann E. Garner. "Effects of music on Alzheimer patients." *Perceptual and Motor Skills* 76, issue 2 (1993): 451–55.

Love, Karen and Jackie Pinkowitz. "Person-centered care for people with dementia: a theoretical and conceptual framework." *Generations Journal of the American Society on Aging* 37, issue 3 (2013): 23–29.

Love, Karen and Jackie Pinkowitz. "The quality chasm: national dementia initiative." *CCAL*. Falls Church, VA (2013). www.daanow.org/dementia-action-alliance/white-paper/.

Mittelman, Mary and Cynthia Epstein. "Meet me: Making art accessible for people with dementia." A study from New York University and the Museum of Modern Art (MoMA). (2009). https://www.moma.org/momaorg/shared/pdfs/docs/meetme/Resources_NYU_Evaluation.pdf.

Perrin, Tessa. "Lifted into a world of rhythm and melody." *Journal of Dementia Care* 6, issue 1 (1998): 22–24.

Pinkowitz, J. and K. Love. "Living Fully with Dementia: Words Matter." Dementia Action Alliance. www.daanow.org/wp-content/uploads/2015/01/Living-Fully-with-Dementia-Words-Matter_9.9.2015.pdf.

Richeson, Nancy E. "Effects of animal-assisted therapy on agitated behaviors and social interactions of older adults with dementia." *American Journal of Alzheimer's Disease & Other Dementia* 18, no. 6 (2003): 353–58.

Roberts, Rosebud. "Hobbies 'improve brain power in old age.'" Mayo Clinic Study. Oct (2013).

Särkämö, Teppo, et al. "Singing is beneficial for memory and mood especially in early dementia." University of Helsinki, Finland. *Journal of Alzheimer's Disease* 49, issue 3 (December 2015).

Schamberger, Magdalena, "Clowning around: Red noses and regeneration," *Bridging Culture and Regeneration,* SURF's online magazine, vol. Winter/Spring 2015, March 2, 2015. http://www.scotregen.co.uk/scotregen/clowning-around-red-noses-and-regeneration/.

Swinnen, Aagje. "Healing words: A study of poetry interventions in dementia care." *Dementia: The International Journal of Social Research and Practice*, November 27, 2014.

Tomaino, Concetta. "Music and the mind: The magical power of sound." *Annals of the New York Academy of Sciences* 1303, no. 1 (2013): 63–79.

Treadaway, Cathy, et al. "Sensor e-Textiles: Designing for persons with late stage dementia." Design4Health International Conference. Sheffield, July (2015).

Treadaway, Cathy et al. "Designing for positive emotion: ludic artefacts to support wellbeing for people with dementia." In *Colors of Care: 9th International Conference on Design and Emotion,* eds Juan Salamanca, Pieter Desmet, Andrés Burbano, et al. (Bogota, Columbia: Design and Emotion Society; Universidad de Los Andes: 2014).

Vidoni, Eric D., Sandra Billinger, Charesa Lee, Jeffrey Burns. "The physical performance test predicts aerobic capacity sufficient for independence in early-stage Alzheimer's." *Journal of Geriatric Physical Therapy* 35, no. 2 (2012): 72–78.

Zeisel, John, with Barry Reisberg, Peter Whitehouse, Robert Woods, and Ad Verheul "Ecopsychosocial Interventions in Cognitive Decline and Dementia: a new terminology and a new paradigm." *American Journal of Alzheimer's Disease and Other Dementias.* (2016).

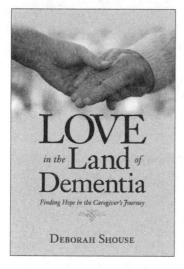

LOVE
in the Land *of*
Dementia:
Finding Hope in the Caregiver's Journey

For many families, a diagnosis of dementia is an ending. For Deborah Shouse, it was a beginning. "My mother taught me how to celebrate and appreciate what we have right now." Through her mother's memory loss, Deborah discovered compassion, moments of quality connection, and deepening love with her mother and other members of her family. *Love in the Land of Dementia* offers insight and hope to family members, friends, and care partners.

Praise for *Love in the Land of Dementia:*

"I have read hundreds of true stories about families dealing with Alzheimer's disease. None were written more wonderfully or truthfully. Readers journey with Deborah Shouse in her superbly written tale, finding hope in the loss and even happiness in the new connection."
—LeAnn Thieman, coauthor of *Chicken Soup for the Caregiver's Soul*

"We have been searching for a text by a family caregiver that we can recommend unreservedly, and now we feel we have found one in *Love in the Land of Dementia.* Whilst never denying the down-turns in caring for

someone with Alzheimer's, Deborah is intelligent and sensitive enough to notice all sorts of things which bring situations alive, give people hope, and constitute treasurable epiphanies."
—John Killick, author of *Dementia Positive*

"There is wisdom in every anecdote, and Deborah Shouse's unique perspective provides caregivers and family members hope and meaning."
—Jeffrey M. Burns, MD, Director of the Alzheimer and Memory Center and Principal Investigator of the Brain Aging Project, University of Kansas Medical Center

"Storytelling is an art, and Deborah Shouse has taken it to a new level. *Love in the Land of Dementia* is a must read for all of us."
—David B. Oliver, PhD, author of *The Human Factor in Nursing Home Care*

Love in the Land of Dementia is insightful, witty, honest, and genuine. This is an excellent book not only for people who have aging parents, but for all those who want to learn about themselves. I highly recommend it."
—Naomi Feil, MSW, ACSW, Executive Director of the Validation Training Institute, author of *V/F Validation: The Feil Method*

"This story has enhanced the way I work with families and is a valuable tool when families and caregivers feel there is no hope left in the disease journey. This book should be mandatory reading for anyone working with a person experiencing dementia."
—Karen Johnson Knappenberger, LMSW, Outreach Coordinator, Alzheimer's Association—Heart of America Chapter

"Each story in *Love in the Land of Dementia* is like an exquisite jewel."
—Victoria Moran, author of *Creating a Charmed Life*